Dr. Kathryn Schrotenboer's Guide to Pregnancy Over 35

Kathryn Schrotenboer, OB/GYN
and Joan Solomon Weiss

Ballantine Books · New York

Library of Congress Catalog Card Number: 84-90808
ISBN: 0-345-31347-X

Manufactured in the United States of America

Cover photo by Don Banks

Book Design by Amy Lamb

FIRST EDITION: MAY 1985

10 9 8 7 6 5 4 3 2 1

To Brian, Michael, Paul, Kristin and Alison

2258101

Acknowledgements

We would like to thank the many women who were willing to share with us their pregnancy experiences and the men who talked with us about the father's role in the childbirth process. We would also like to thank Drs. Joan Handler, Linda Kestenbaum and Barbara Gordon for their insights into the psychological aspects of pregnancy. Finally we would like to thank Ms. Lori Woods for her help in the research involved in this book.

Table of Contents

Dr. Kathryn Schrotenboer's Guide to Pregnancy Over 35

Is It Too Late?

Ellen walked into Kathryn's office, a decade after her first childbirth experience, pregnant again. She was 28 then. She is 38 now, and more anxious than she was the first time. She expressed her concerns to the doctor: "Now that I'm older, how can I make it through the pregnancy? Won't it be complicated? Won't I be sick? Won't there be something wrong with the baby?"

Ellen's concerns are quite common among women who are expectant mothers after the "expected" time. That "expected" time has expanded recently to include women in their early thirties. Today it is considered quite acceptable for women to wait until after their thirtieth birthday to start a family or to add a second or third child to a family started in their twenties. But if you get pregnant after age 35, especially if it's to have your first baby, you probably won't escape the observation that you're too old for this sort of thing. Your mother may say, "You're too old to be a mother—and I'm much too old to be a grandmother." Or an aunt, a cousin, or a friend tells you how difficult your pregnancy will be, how impossible the birth, how high your chances are of having a less-than-perfect baby. You may even be warned that you'll lack the patience for the demands of infant care, that you'll hate being tied down. If you are fortunate enough to have the support of your family and friends, and to be confident in your decision, you may find that your doctor does not share your optimism. Some physicians automatically consider women over 35 to be "high-risk" maternity patients, and make their "prejudices" quite clear. Whether these notions are held by physician or by friend, that is exactly what they are—prejudices. Such outdated beliefs raise more obstacles to a safe, normal pregnancy and birth than a woman's age can.

As we'll soon see, your age will most likely not be an obstacle to a healthy childbirth experience, nor to your capacity to be a good mother. Older mothers, with the experience of their years behind them, are likely to be more patient and tolerant in the parenting role. They have already done many of the things they have set out to do. The baby is a planned addition to their lives, not an unwelcome intruder who will rob them of their youth and their dreams. Those of you who have waited so long to fulfill the dream of a family can develop into mothers who are second to none.

As an obstetrician associated with New York Hospital, Kathryn sees many over-35 women on the brink of motherhood. Most of them are going through normal, healthy pregnancies, though many, like Ellen, bring with them concerns about their age. Am I too old for a safe pregnancy? Will I have a healthy baby? How will my years as a career woman affect my ability to be a mother?

Although Kathryn was under 35 when she had her own babies (28 when she gave birth to her son and 31 when she delivered twin girls), she was already entrenched in her medical career, and shared some of those same concerns. Is it possible to be a good doctor *and* a good mother? Coauthor Joan was a well-established writer by the time she gave birth (she had one son at age 29 and the other at 31), and also had the concerns of a career woman embarking on a new and very different kind of career.

Although pregnancy for women over 35 is not as different as most women would imagine, there are differences, both physical and emotional, that made the authors feel that this kind of book is a needed resource to the "older" pregnant woman. And they felt that their professional and personal experience made them the ideal team to write this book. As a female obstetrician, Kathryn knows what it's like both to experience pregnancy herself and to help hundreds of other women achieve a healthy pregnancy and childbirth. And because of the location of her practice—in a major urban center—many of those women are over 35. She has heard them talk about the prejudices they've encountered from both family members and physicians. This book will help to dispel such prejudice by countering it with accurate and useful information.

As Joan and Kathryn looked at childbirth statistics, they realized just how many women would benefit from pregnancy information tailored to this over-35 age group. For despite society's prejudices, more and more "older" women are bucking those attitudes and getting pregnant anyway. In 1981, more than 170,000 women had babies despite their "advanced" age of 35-plus. The trend for more than a decade now has been for women to delay parenthood until their early or even their late thirties. Government statistics indicate how strong a trend it is. From 1972 to 1981, the rate of first births to women from 35 to 39 years of age increased by 56%. (In that same time span, the rate of first births for women in their lower twenties actually decreased, and for women in their upper twenties the rate increased by only a third.) Many "older" mothers don't stop at one child. Their rate of second births also increased during that same period, by a sizable 45%. The twenties are still the decade of life in which most women have their babies, but for an increasingly large group of women, it is at least a decade too soon.

Why are women waiting longer to become mothers? In 1970, three out of every twenty women aged 25 to 29 were unmarried; by 1980, that figure had doubled to six out of twenty. As women continue to postpone marriage, and as divorce rates make increasing inroads into marriage rates, the birth statistics are reflecting the changing realities of family life. It is less common now for children to be conceived to hold together a failing marriage; women today prefer to start their families only in stable marital situations.

The over-35 woman who is currently having babies is typically a well-educated, middle-class woman who has spent many years building up her career and is now, finally, ready for a child. The advent of birth control has made it possible for her to plan her years in that way: first a career, when that was most important to her, and now a baby, before her years for having a baby run out.

That is often the impetus for having a child at this stage of life—the fear that this is the last opportunity to make such a decision, the thought that motherhood must be now, or be never. Once you pass your 35th birthday, 40 doesn't seem so far away, and neither does the end of fertility. If you have not previously felt ready for a baby, you may now embrace the possibility of parenthood. Or you may feel a void where there should be a child. Your career is no longer satisfying or no longer enough. You want to explore the nurturing side of you that has been hidden under your rigorous professionalism. You want to have a baby, and you want to have it now.

The Fertility Question

You may worry that you have waited too long, that now that you want a baby, you may have trouble conceiving. The possibility of infertility is a real issue to women who wait until their mid- or late thirties or their forties to try to conceive. Many of Kathryn's patients bring it up to her, especially if they've tried for a few months to become pregnant without success. Although some studies do point to a decided decline in fertility in women over 30, some experts believe that they exaggerate the frequency of fertility problems. For example, John Bongaarts, senior associate of the Center for Policy Studies, the Population Council, says that only an estimated 19.7% of women aged 35 to 40 are permanently infertile.[1]

Why are there risks at all? Why do the years bring with them reduced fertility, whether it is the sharp drop that some scientists claim or the more gradual decline that others see? One of the causes of infertility that can strike women of any age, endometriosis, is more prevalent in older, childless women. In this condition, tissue similar to that lining the uterus is found attached to other pelvic organs, such as the ovaries or the fallopian tubes. Even a slight degree of endometriosis may interfere with tubal function and with the motion of the egg down the tube; a more severe case may involve complete blockage of the tubes. Fertility is often compromised in women with this disease. Since pregnancy helps to prevent it from occurring, women who put off pregnancy are more likely to develop it, and then to have trouble getting pregnant when they choose to.

1. The infertility issue was highlighted recently by a French study, published in *The New England Journal of Medicine* in 1982, which involved the artificial insemination of more than 2,000 women who had borne no previous children. Within a twelve-cycle period of insemination, only 53.6% of the women over 35 became pregnant; that figure compared, unfavorably, with the success rate of 73% for women under 25, 74.1% for the 26 to 30 age group, and 61.5% for women aged 31 to 35.

Sexually transmitted genital infections such as chlamydia and mycoplasma can also compromise fertility, and are tested for in infertility workups. They may be present in a man or a woman for a long time without causing any apparent symptoms. But a woman may experience pelvic inflammatory disease—an infection of the uterus, ovaries, and tubes that can cause tubal scarring—or the man may experience nonspecific urethritis or be found to have a lowered sperm count. An "older" woman, who has had more sexual partners, is more likely to show evidence of these infections. Pelvic inflammatory disease may have developed in other ways, through the use of an intrauterine device, for example, or through gonorrheal infection. Again, an older woman has had more years in which such a condition might have developed.

Another possible reason for reduced fertility with age involves what's known as a "luteal phase defect." In this condition, the corpus luteum, a small cyst in the ovary that produces hormones to support the early pregnancy, is not functioning properly. If the corpus luteum is deficient in its hormone production, the hormonal milieu of the uterus does not support proper implantation of the fertilized egg. This condition seems to be more common in over-35 women.

Although this information may seem discouraging to you, there is really every reason for optimism because of advances in infertility management. A luteal phase defect can be treated with medication once the condition is discovered. Endometriosis has been found to be quite responsive to hormonal management, and is *not* a sentence to a childless future. A chlamydia infection may be treated with antibiotics. Pelvic scarring from past pelvic inflammatory disease can often be successfully treated through surgery, the extent of the disease dictating the complexity of the operative procedure. New advances in test tube fertilization may lead to successes in the future for women who previously failed with conventional fertility treatments. Infertility can be frustrating, but it is not necessarily forever.

By waiting until your midthirties or later to try to start a family, you may have somewhat reduced your chances of success—but the chances for parenthood are still in your favor. It may take you somewhat longer than it would have a decade ago, but isn't a baby worth the wait? Besides, the wait is not likely to be interminable. According to a study of 792 first pregnancies, the median time for conception was two months for women from 15 to 25 years of age and 3.8 months for the 35 to 44 age group. So if you tend toward the average, you can be expecting to hold your baby in your arms in little more than a year from the time you begin your efforts to conceive. One point to remember is to keep making those efforts regularly, at least three or four times during the week that ovulation is occurring. (Ovulation occurs fourteen days before the beginning of menstruation. If you're on a twenty-eight-day cycle, for example, it occurs on the fourteenth day of the cycle. If you're on a thirty-two-day cycle, it occurs on the eighteenth day.) Some scientists point to a decline in coital frequency as a prime reason for the lower conception rates of older couples. If you do have trouble getting pregnant, do not wait too long before seeking medical assistance. If you do not conceive after six months of trying, you and your mate should consult with a physician. You're not too old now to become pregnant, but you don't want to wait until it *is* too late.

Exploding the Myths, Facing the Facts

Whether conceiving is easy or arduous for you, you may fear a rough road ahead. In this book, Joan and Kathryn will examine how unfounded many of those fears are, and how an over-35 pregnancy can run as smooth a course as any. Age alone does not undermine the pregnancy process, though it does introduce some additional concerns, which will be explored in depth in subsequent chapters. One legitimate concern involves the increasing incidence of genetic disorders in the offspring of older mothers. Fortunately, this problem can largely be prevented through the use of a medical technique known as amniocentesis. This book contains a detailed description not only of the technique itself but what it's like to go through amniocentesis. (See pages 104-24.)

What about other complications of pregnancy? Are you more vulnerable to toxemia of pregnancy, to diabetic difficulties, to Rh problems, to placental malformations, to all the other things you've heard can go wrong during the period of fetal development? *Dr. Kathryn Schrotenboer's Guide to Pregnancy Over 35* will explore just which pregnancy complications are age-related, which women are the most vulnerable, and how the difficulties can best be prevented or overcome. A woman of any age who was healthy before the pregnancy will likely stay healthy throughout it, and deliver a healthy baby. Only a woman who suffers from a chronic health problem—more common with increasing age—will be more apt to experience a difficult pregnancy. But because of great strides made in prenatal diagnosis and care, the odds are that even she can surmount the difficulties and go on to have a perfectly normal child.

One feature of pregnancy that may be different for an over-35 woman is the childbirth experience itself. An older mother has a higher probability of delivering surgically rather than vaginally. Some of the reasons for the higher Cesarean rate, as we'll discuss later, are legitimate, while others result from misconceptions. Cesarean birth will be explained in depth in this book—including ways to avoid an unnecessary Cesarean, what to expect if it is necessary in your case, and ways to recover from the disappointment that often accompanies the Cesarean experience. (See pages 192-211.)

As you begin your pregnancy, you'll need to adjust your lifestyle to the demands of your changing body. You may be used to giving your professional pursuits top priority and spending your leisure time doing what you want to do, whether it's playing tennis, skiing, theater-going, or vacationing in lands half a globe away. But you may see this lifestyle slipping away with each passing month of the pregnancy, and you may fear it will never return once your baby is born. The adjustment can be difficult, but you *can* embrace the new without entirely giving up the old. Having a baby does mean change, it even means loss, but what is gained through the experience of childbearing and child-rearing is much greater than what is given up.

At the age of 35 or older, your experience of pregnancy and childbirth can be as positive and rewarding as it is for any other woman. *Dr. Kathryn Schrotenboer's Guide to Pregnancy Over 35* will guide you through each stage and concern of your pregnancy. It will address your special concerns: your nutritional requirements, the sports you should or shouldn't be playing, your sexual life. It will arm you with the information to help you make intelligent decisions about the pregnancy as well as the birth, and it will help you get through the *other* side of the childbirth experience, when the baby is at hand. This book will also help you deal with the emotional side of pregnancy and give you an understanding of the emotions your mate may be going through, even if he seems stoic through it all. Most important, this book provides the reassurance that it is *not* too late for you to have a baby. In fact, you bring a lot of qualities to the experience that are often lacking in younger women—maturity, patience, a sense of competence, a firm grasp on your own identity. If you choose, carefully and deliberately, to have your baby at this time in your life, if you feel finally ready to experience one of life's greatest challenges and greatest joys, then you couldn't choose a better time.

1

Your Medical Care Options: Finding the Right Person and the Right Place

The decision to have a baby was a hard enough one to make at this time in your life. Now you're faced with another set of choices— who should help you bring your baby into the world, and where should that great event take place? Because those choices will set the tone for your whole childbearing experience, they should be made thoughtfully and deliberately. This is the opportunity for you and your mate to participate fully in the decisions regarding the pregnancy and birth. Once you've made the decision that's right for you and your family, you'll be secure in knowing that the health-care aspects of childbirth will be handled by a person you can trust in an environment that suits your needs.

The options vary depending on where you live. In some areas there is little choice. The only facility for childbirth may be the community hospital, and there might be only a few doctors to choose from. But even in small towns and rural areas, more alternatives are beginning to emerge, as a midwife may set up practice, or an alternative birth center may open its doors. In large cities, of course, the choice of facilities and physicians is far greater. Wherever you live, you and your partner will want to explore the range of options early in your pregnancy or even before you conceive.

Selecting the Place

One of your most important considerations is the setting in which you wish to deliver your baby. Although the vast majority of women give birth in a hospital, there are variations even within the hospital environment that you should be aware of. And there are out-of-hospital alternatives that are becoming more popular, particularly in the western part of the country.

To gather information about a particular facility, you can either talk to a doctor who is affiliated with that institution or call up the department of obstetrics. You might also want to ask whether you and your husband can be taken on a tour of its maternity facilities; many hospitals are willing to arrange for this. You'll learn what the hospital's setup is for labor and delivery—what the labor room is like; whether you'll stay there for the delivery; whether you'll deliver in the same bed you labor in. You'll also notice what the general atmosphere and the decor is like. Many people choose a hospital based mostly on that consideration: What are the rooms like? Are there curtains on the windows? How cheery does it all seem? It is certainly a plus for a hospital to have a pleasant atmosphere, but it is not as important as having solid diagnostic equipment and the availability of top emergency physicians. Some of the country's outstanding university hospitals are in old buildings that you would *never* choose for the look of their rooms or for their food. In choosing a hospital, consider the question of safety before that of beauty.

There may be other issues of importance to you that you should raise at this point in your pregnancy. You may want to ask hospital personnel whether the father is allowed at a delivery, including a Cesarean, and how liberal are his opportunities for visiting after the birth. Most hospitals do allow fathers to be present for the labor and birth and even to participate in some fashion. Most fathers, given the opportunity, do choose to be present, though others pass up the chance. (This is not a reason to judge a man harshly. He may simply feel that he will be more of a hindrance than a help, and save his participation for after the birth.)

You may also want to find out whether there is a "family" time after the delivery for parents and baby to be together. If you have other children, it may be important for you to know if they'll be allowed to see you and the baby soon after the birth, and visit you in the hospital during your stay there. Other common and relevant questions involve a hospital's rooming-in policy—just how much time during the day will you be able to have your baby in your room with you? And how supportive is the hospital of a mother's desire to breast-feed—will the baby be brought to you often enough to start off the nursing experience in the best possible way? Feel free to ask any other questions you may have about the labor, the delivery, and your stay in the hospital (including its length and its cost). In that way, you and your mate will be able to make a fully informed choice about the place in which you'll have your baby. Even if you are already set on a particular hospital because it's the one your physician is affiliated with—and you don't want to change your physician—it's still a good idea to take a tour of its delivery and maternity wings and ask the questions that are important to you. By investigating ahead, you'll know what to expect, and won't be upset by the unknown at the time of the birth.

There is one question that more and more expectant parents are asking of hospital administrators and physicians: Under what circumstances is fetal monitoring used on laboring women? It's a question *you* might want to ask before you settle on a hospital. This procedure involves the use of ultrasound, or a tiny electrode attached to the baby's scalp to detect the fetal heartbeat, and a strap around the mother's abdomen (or a thin plastic tube within the uterus) to detect contractions during labor. The use of ultrasound has been brought into question because, although there is absolutely no evidence that ultrasound exposure has any adverse effects on the fetus, it cannot be *proven* to be safe. Critics have also suggested that doctors rush to do Cesarean deliveries at the first sign of an irregular or slow heartbeat revealed by the monitor. There may have been some truth to that allegation in the early years of fetal monitoring, but with increased knowledge and growing understanding of the patterns of the fetal heartbeat, a Cesarean is less likely to be done out of misinformation or unwarranted concern. There are now tests that elicit additional information should the fetal heartbeat decrease. The major one involves taking a blood sample from the fetal scalp and checking its pH (acidity level). That measurement indicates how much oxygen the baby is receiving and whether or not it's under stress. There are also procedures performed, such as administering oxygen to the mother, or changing her position (perhaps from one side to the other or putting her head down and feet up) to improve the situation should the monitoring indicate a problem. At New York Hospital/Cornell Medical Center and at many other major medical centers, women are routinely put on a fetal monitor during labor. Such a practice offers them the highest degree of safety, as the patterns of the fetal heartbeat and the uterine contractions can be observed on a continuous basis. Many women find it reassuring to hear the heartbeat and to know that things are going well; as an added benefit, the contraction is visible on the monitor before the woman feels it, so her Lamaze coach can prepare her for what's about to happen.

Whether you prefer a hospital setting or a less formal environment, we recommend looking over all the options. The following discussion will help to familiarize you with the alternatives available to you for your childbirth, the advantages and disadvantages of the various facilities, and how to choose among them.

In-Hospital Births: If you are concerned primarily with safety, hospitals are your best choice. They are most likely to have the personnel and equipment to handle emergencies that can arise in even a seemingly low-risk pregnancy. If an infection develops, or hemorrhage, or other uncommon but possible complications, a modern hospital facility will be able to treat you promptly and properly. If the baby develops a problem in its first day or two of life, appropriate treatment is more available in a hospital setting than in alternative birth facilities. Some women, however, think of hospitals as cold, sterile places. But as forbidding as a hospital may seem, its mission is to preserve life; it is the safest place in which to deliver a baby, though possibly not the most "natural."

If you decide on a hospital delivery, you may also have another decision to make: which hospital to deliver in? In most fair-sized communities there is more than one to choose from, and in large cities there may be more than a score. Ask about the presence of emergency facilities, such as a blood bank and an operating room, the availability of anesthesia on a twenty-four-hour basis, the availability of a pediatrician, particularly one who specializes in birth problems, and the presence of an intensive care unit for sick babies. Large medical centers are more likely to be fully equipped for both normal and complicated births, and to have first-class laboratory facilities and diagnostic equipment. As more sophisticated ways are being developed to deal with difficult deliveries and sick babies, the greater the advantage of being in a facility that can apply the new techniques.

But many smaller communities have only relatively small hospitals, generally fine facilities for most women and their new babies. Some people who have a wide choice of facilities choose a small hospital because they prefer its more relaxed, homey atmosphere. If a problem arises that these hospitals can't handle, they try to transport the woman before the birth, by ambulance or by helicopter, to the nearest large medical center; if events have proceeded too quickly for that, and the birth has occurred, they will transport the baby who is in trouble. Women who plan to deliver at such community hospitals should ask ahead of time about the arrangements for transfer should a serious complication develop. If you anticipate a normal, uncomplicated delivery, and know that emergency transport is available, the choice of a small community hospital can be a sound one for you. If this is your case, ask the same questions you would of a larger hospital in regard to a blood bank, an operating room, anesthesia, and the availability of a pediatrician; make your inquiries of a doctor or other caregiver associated with the hospital. Find out what the hospital's reputation is in the community. There may well be a sound basis for its medical standing.

Alternative Birth Centers within Hospitals: Hospitals are known for providing a safe but often emotionally sterile birth experience; some are trying to improve their images without compromising safety by forming alternative birth centers within their facilities. Usually located on the labor floor, such centers are designed to accommodate the family during labor and delivery. Much of the woman's hospital experience occurs within a "birthing room"—a room more like a bedroom than a labor room. It's designed to be as homelike as possible, with curtains and carpets, plants and pictures, a comfortable bed, and other reminders of home. The woman labors there and gives birth there, most often with her mate at her side to share in this awesome experience and to help coach her and comfort her. Other aspects of these alternative birth centers differ greatly from hospital to hospital. Anesthesia may or may not be made available, for example, depending on the center. In some birthing rooms fetal monitors and intravenous hookups are standard equipment; in others, they are rarely or never used. The option of alternative birth centers within hospitals is growing increasingly popular as more women want a natural experience without endangering themselves or their baby in any way; in this "home" within a hospital they can feel relaxed and at ease, confident that if anything goes wrong they can be transferred immediately to the regular delivery wing to receive emergency care. If this sounds like the ideal arrangement for you, you may have to do some legwork to find the right situation. Hospitals generally don't allow high-risk patients to use their birthing rooms, and some hospitals automatically define women over 35 as high risk. So you may have to query a few hospitals before you find one that will accept you in its alternative birth center. If you *do* have a problem pregnancy (and being over 35 does not in itself mean that you do), then such a center is not the place for you.

Sometimes an alternative birth center within a hospital or directly adjacent to one is run by an independent childbirth group. As long as it is easily accessible to hospital facilities and emergency facilities, that's fine. It's when such centers are not physically part of a hospital that problems can arise because of the time it takes to transfer emergency patients.

Hospital Clinics: If you cannot afford private obstetrical care in a first-rate hospital, you do not have to sacrifice a safe hospital birth. Many hospitals run obstetrical clinics at a moderate cost, and some of them are excellent. If you're interested in this option, find out whether you will be assigned to a particular doctor or will see a different doctor at each visit. Ask whether the doctor who will deliver you will be one you will have met during your pregnancy. And find out how long the typical prenatal visit lasts. Some clinics rush their patients through, while others give each patient sufficient time. If you know anyone who's been a patient at a particular clinic, ask what her experience there has been.

Your experience as a clinic patient will be different from the experience of a private patient in that you'll probably be attended to by interns and residents. Their work will be done under the supervision of physicians affiliated with the hospital, and the medical quality will usually be quite high. You may not have as much privacy as you would like, or as much individual attention, but in clinics associated with university teaching hospitals, your health and your baby's health should not be compromised.

Out-of-Hospital Births: Alternative Birth Centers away from hospitals are similar to those inside hospitals in that they provide a more homelike setting for the delivery and a more natural birth experience than does the typical hospital. They also emphasize family presence and participation, including not only the father but often the siblings as well. Either a physician or a nurse-midwife with physician backup in case of emergency may attend the delivery. The costs are lower than in a hospital and the stay shorter—in most cases, mother and baby go home within twelve hours of the delivery. All these features make this type of center an attractive birth environment for many women—more natural than a hospital birth, safer than a home birth. These centers try to build in safety in a variety of ways, including the careful screening of the women they accept in their programs. Common reasons for nonacceptance include a past Cesarean delivery, a physical illness such as cardiac disease or diabetes, as well as the physical state of being "too old." In this context, "too old" often means being 35 or over for a first baby, or 40 or over for a subsequent baby. So even if you are interested in these centers for your birth experience, they may not want to admit you because of your age.

The vast majority of women who give birth at alternative birth centers have a positive and safe experience. The labor and delivery process goes smoothly, and the whole family can take joy in the miracle of birth. But in a small percentage of cases things don't go so well, and the center is not prepared to deal with the difficulty. There is no equipment or personnel on hand to do an emergency Cesarean delivery; there is no immediate and effective way to deal with hemorrhage; there is usually no pediatrician on hand to minister to a baby born with a serious problem. These centers generally do have arrangements with nearby hospitals to accept their patients who get into trouble, and arrangements with ambulance companies for quick transport. The drawback is that "nearby" is sometimes not near enough. If the placenta starts to separate, or if an amniotic fluid embolism forms (a soft mass of amniotic fluid that can travel to the lungs), quick treatment is crucial. If a woman begins to hemorrhage after delivery, she can bleed heavily enough to die within five minutes. If a baby is not breathing, an ambulance ride of half an hour or even just ten minutes can spell untold damage to the infant, and even death. While alternative birth centers provide safe birth settings for most women, they are simply not well enough equipped or staffed to handle all emergencies. And despite their careful screening of patients, it's impossible to know for sure when an emergency will occur. The safer alternative is to choose a center within or physically adjacent to a hospital, or a nurse-midwife program connected with a hospital (described later in this chapter).

Home Births: More than fifty years ago, births started shifting from home to hospital for reasons of medical safety. In the past decade, some women have decided that the old ways are better, and are delivering their babies at home. They are doing it because they want a birth environment that is not just homelike, but actually is home. And they want their family and even friends to participate in this great event.

The home birth movement is growing more popular; in Oregon, for example, about 5% of births occur at home. But by choosing this method, you may be putting yourself and your baby at risk. You cannot know ahead of time, with absolute certainty, that yours will not be a complicated birth. In a small percentage of cases—about one or two percent—a serious complication *will* occur. It can lead to the death of the mother, or death or mental retardation of the infant. In a home environment, the chances for preventing or properly treating these emergency situations are vastly reduced. The position of the American College of Obstetricians and Gynecologists, as put forth in this policy statement, is that home births present unacceptable risks: "Labor and delivery, while a physiologic process, clearly presents potential hazards to both mother and fetus before and after birth. These hazards require standards of safety which are provided in the hospital setting and cannot be matched in the home situation." Kathryn's position, also, is that no woman, either under or over 35, should even consider giving birth at home.

Selecting the Person

The decision about your birth environment has another vital component: Who should provide for your health care during your pregnancy and perform the delivery? If you already see an obstetrician-gynecologist for checkups and for any gynecological problems you may have, this part of your decision may be an easy one.

If you're happy with your doctor, if you share an easy rapport and are confident in his or her skills, that might be the ideal person for you. But make sure your physician actually *does* deliver babies. And ask what childbirth facility he or she is affiliated with. If your doctor is skilled and respected in the field, the likelihood is that the hospital will be a fine one. But it's a good idea for you to take a tour of its maternity facilities anyway, and of any alternative birth center on its premises, if that option interests you.

If you don't currently use an obstetrician-gynecologist, or are dissatisfied with the one you do use, then your task will be somewhat harder. First, you'll want to familiarize yourself with the types of health-care personnel who perform deliveries. Obstetrician-gynecologists are the specialists in this area of medicine. They have gone through many years of education and training, and are fully prepared to handle both routine and complicated births, including Cesarean deliveries. They are ready to act quickly and effectively in case of an emergency. Most of these physicians have been certified by the American Board of Obstetrics and Gynecology; some younger physicians may be board-eligible but not yet certified because they haven't been in practice long enough to take the examination. Even an older doctor may not be certified yet if he or she has started up practice slowly or taken prior training in another specialty.

Another possible choice of doctor is the family practitioner. Some of these physicians practice obstetrics in addition to their other work. They usually have not had as extensive a training in obstetrics as have specialists, but they may be very practiced in delivering babies and perfectly capable of handling normal births. If you're considering using such a doctor, ask what his or her training in obstetrics has been, and what kind of backup will be available in case of an emergency. An obstetrician should be immediately available to handle complications, particularly if a Cesarean birth is required. (Most family practitioners do not perform Cesarean deliveries.)

Yet another alternative is a nurse-midwife. These health practitioners offer a birth experience that is somewhat different, and particularly appealing to women who want another woman to guide them through this womanly experience. (Currently, the majority of obstetricians are male and the majority of nurse-midwives female.) Their emphasis is strongly on nonintervention, and on providing as natural an experience as possible. Typically, they spend a great deal of time with each patient during the pregnancy period, and offer her constant support and comfort while she is in labor. Many obstetricians are impressed with the gentle, encouraging manner of midwives, and try to bring some of that attitude to their own laboring patients. It's important to remember, however, that nurse-midwives—professionals with nursing degrees as well as specialized intensive training in midwifery—are *not* as well trained as are obstetricians, particularly in the treatment of complications. As part of their training they are taught to recognize complications, and to call in a physician when medical intervention may be necessary.

If you decide that you would like the more natural type of birth that a midwife provides, it's important that the birth take place in a facility where medical supervision is available. A number of hospitals now have nurse-midwife programs for women who prefer that option; that is a sound way to achieve a birth that's safe and as natural as your situation allows. Some nurse-midwives work in teams with doctors, perhaps in a partnership situation or as members of a group practice. They may alternate days on call, with the doctor available should complications arise. These many variations offer you a great deal of choice in shaping your childbearing experience.

There are also practitioners known as lay midwives who supervise pregnancies and deliver babies. The testing and licensing requirements for them vary widely from state to state, and in some states it is not legal for them to practice. Some lay midwives are well trained, and quite capable of handling normal births. But some learn the profession simply by observing a few births, and without any special training or testing label themselves midwives and go into the delivery business. If you consider using a lay midwife, check the midwife's licensing, training, and experience carefully. You don't want to put yourself and your baby into the wrong hands.

Once you narrow down your decision to the type of health professional you prefer, you still have to choose the particular person who will guide you through the health aspects of your pregnancy and deliver your baby. If you're not satisfied with your current obstetrician-gynecologist, that means getting one or more recommendations and checking them out. One excellent source of recommendations is a doctor you are already using, such as your family doctor or pediatrician. That physician is familiar with your personality and perhaps your health history, and can use that knowledge to make an informed referral. If you spell out exactly what you are looking for in an obstetrician, you're likely to be quite satisfied with your current doctor's recommendation. Another method is to choose the hospital or other facility in which you'd like to deliver your baby, and then inquire of its department of obstetrics or nurse-midwifery program for the name of affiliated professionals. Asking friends for a recommendation is not exactly a scientific way of going about finding a doctor, but it works for a lot of people. The trick is not to ask the friend if she "liked" her doctor—her taste, preferences, and needs may be very different from yours—but to ask specific questions about the doctor's practice and approach to delivering babies. Then you will be able to use her experience as a useful guideline in choosing the professional who will best meet your needs.

Doctors Alone, Doctors in Groups: Increasingly, you'll find that the doctors and even the nurse-midwives who are recommended to you are in group practices, and you'll have to decide whether that's an arrangement that will work for you, or whether you prefer a solo practitioner. Both these types of practices have advantages and disadvantages for you to consider. Women who choose a single practitioner generally like the individual attention they receive and the personal relationship they develop with their doctor. It's nice to know that you'll be seeing the same person visit after visit, and that this person you know well will in all likelihood be the one who will deliver your baby. If your doctor becomes ill or goes on a vacation during your pregnancy, you will probably be referred to a trusted colleague. Since there's an outside chance that this second doctor will perform your delivery, it's a good idea to have at least one of your prenatal visits with that physician. In that way, if it's the second doctor who is there when the time comes, you'll be sure to know the man or woman behind the mask.

Because of the busy schedules of most obstetricians, some of them have banded together in group practices to increase their efficiency and to reduce the tremendous demands on their time. Their patients can benefit from this efficiency, and from the somewhat more relaxed pace that results. The doctor is less likely to

be overtired and overworked. Appointments are less likely to be
canceled, as the office can still be covered while some patients are
in labor. And the doctors who are with those patients in labor
don't have to be concerned about getting back quickly to an office
full of waiting patients. But what a woman has to give up, to some
extent, is the personal relationship with a single doctor. Although
one of the physicians may be her primary one, she is likely to see
the other physicians on some of her prenatal visits. In addition,
she has little assurance that her primary doctor will be the one to
deliver her baby.

If you are considering a group practice for your obstetrical care,
there are some issues you should straighten out from the start.
Find out how the group works—for example, does each doctor
have his or her own patients, and just cover others for vacations
or weekends? Or do they split up the week and cover alternate
days? Or do they divide the workload in some other way? Some
group schedules may fit in better with your particular needs and
preferences. It would also be helpful if you could find out whether
the members of the group have similar attitudes and values in
regard to managing pregnancies and deliveries, and whether they
approach the practice of medicine in essentially the same way.

Asking the Questions, Understanding the Answers: As women are
becoming more active medical consumers, and taking a partnership
role in their medical care (including their obstetrical management),
the practice of interviewing obstetricians has become more popular. Kathryn has been on the receiving end of many such an
interview. The principle of finding out about a doctor before making a selection is a good one, and it often works out well. There
is some general information you *should* seek very early on, at an
interview or at a first visit. You should ask, for example, about a
doctor's fees, what they will include, how often the billing will
take place, and whether insurance payments will be accepted. Usually the amount of the fee and the billing practices do not vary
widely within a certain geographical area, but this is still information that should be obtained before making a final decision.
You should find out whether the doctor has telephone hours, whether
there's a backup during vacation periods, and what the procedure
is for an emergency. You should, of course, inquire about the
physician's hospital affiliation, and try to arrange the type of hos-

pital tour described earlier in this chapter. You might also wish to ask whether the doctor welcomes the husband's attendance at regular prenatal appointments and at the birth itself.

Another avenue of questioning should deal with delivery practices—most importantly, what is the doctor's attitude toward natural childbirth, since it is important that the doctor's practices in this regard mesh with your preferences. If you want as natural a childbirth as possible, you'll want to know that you'll have your doctor's support and encouragement in this, and that drugs will not be pressed on you unless you're sure you want them. On the other hand, if you prefer to take some medication to reduce your pain, it's important to know that your doctor will agree to give you some, and won't make you feel like a "failure" for your request.

You'll also want to know how many women over 35 are seen in the obstetrics part of the practice, and what the physician's attitude is toward childbearing at this "older" end of the spectrum. Physicians who treat few pregnant women in their midthirties and older may be reluctant to take on "older" patients and may treat them very differently than they do younger women. Certainly, attention should be given to a woman's age. But her treatment should be based on the normal, not on the abnormal, and nothing should automatically be done differently based on her age alone. As one major example, she should not be scheduled for a Cesarean delivery simply because she's over 35—but some physicians with limited experience in dealing with older pregnant women might do just that.

There are other advantages to be gained by meeting with a doctor before you make your final choice. You'll learn something about the doctor's personality, about the rapport you two have together, and about the trust you feel in his or her medical judgment. You may discover that the type of care you want is totally *different* from the care you'll get with this doctor. For example, if the most important considerations for you are that you do not want fetal monitoring, or an episiotomy, or an enema, and that you do want to give birth in bed and then go home within three hours, the doctor may feel uncomfortable caring for you and would refer you to a nurse-midwife program where you would be happier.

There are also drawbacks to interviewing physicians that you should be aware of. The answers you get may not always provide you with the information you're seeking. If you ask the physician, for example, how many babies are delivered each year in the practice, the answer will be hard to interpret. If the number is high—maybe 200 or even 300 a year per doctor—that can be an indication that the physician is overworked, and likely to give you short shrift, *or* a clue that he or she is sought after on the basis of impressive medical skills. A doctor with a good reputation is likely to deliver a lot of babies. If the number of deliveries is a low one, perhaps thirty a year or less, you may feel that you'll get plenty of the doctor's time, but wonder if that time is worth it if the doctor's practice is comparatively so small. Another common question is the percentage of Cesarean births a doctor performs. Here, too, the answer can be misleading. If the percentage cited seems high, it can indicate either that the doctor is too quick to perform Cesareans or that the practice includes a large number of high-risk patients.

In other instances, also, answers can confuse or mislead you. As the questions tend to be mostly hypothetical ones, the answers cannot completely predict a doctor's actual behavior in a delivery situation. When the questions are put in the form of demands, they can start the doctor-patient relationship off on the wrong foot. The best tactic is to ask those questions that will provide you with substantial, definitive information, such as fees, the age range of patients, emergency availability, and the use of drugs during labor and delivery. In discussing other issues, such as the performance of episiotomies and the use of fetal monitoring, it's helpful to evaluate just how open the doctor is in explaining his or her views and ways of practicing. They may not always be the views you started out with, but you may come to see the medical rationale of the physician's decisions. The most important thing is that your questions are answered fully and clearly, and that there's an open line of communication between you and the doctor. You should feel comfortable and at ease during your meeting, and have the sense that the doctor understands your values in terms of how they affect the childbirth experience. It is also important that you figure out just which medical practices matter most to you, and which are of secondary significance. For example, if you are generally satisfied with a doctor's expertise and approach, but not happy that you will be shaved before delivery or given an enema, you may decide that that's a small price to pay for excellent care. If you develop a comfortable relationship with the doctor, you may discover that there's some flexibility in aspects of your maternity care, and that your input will make a difference in how you are treated.

Changing Doctors: Some women, instead of interviewing a number of doctors, start seeing a doctor through a referral if their initial impression is a good one. In that way, they are judging a doctor on actual medical behavior as well as personality characteristics, not solely on performance in an interview situation. However a doctor is chosen, it is your option to change doctors if your expectations are not being met. If a doctor doesn't answer your questions forthrightly and completely, or doesn't return your phone calls, those are good reasons to look elsewhere. This is not the time in your life to settle for second best. You have every right to medical care that is both responsible and responsive. If you've made a mistake with your first choice, and your doctor is not all that you thought, there's no harm in your trying again, this time with some experience behind you. There is a place and a person that's right for you.

2

Your Pregnant Body: How You'll Look, How You'll Feel

When you try to picture how pregnancy will affect you, you might focus on an image of yourself waddling into the bathroom to take care of your early morning sickness. But beyond the awkwardness and the nausea commonly associated with pregnancy, there are myriad changes affecting virtually every part and every system of a pregnant woman's body. Some of them are glaringly apparent, such as the bulging abdomen and the blossoming breasts and the different way of walking. Others are hidden to view, the ones involving circulatory and respiratory and digestive adjustments to the state of expectant motherhood. For these nine months, you're going to look and feel differently than you did before and will after. Your body is forming and nurturing new life, and your life will be different during this time of creation.

There are so many changes to undergo, you may wonder how you will manage to cope with them all. Can your over-35 body stand the strain? Can you stand the discomfort? If you're healthy and in good physical shape to begin with, your age does *not* mean that you will have a difficult or particularly uncomfortable pregnancy. To hear it from women who have been through it is to know that your "advanced" age doesn't have to work against you. Says one pregnant 38-year-old, "After hearing so many negative stories about pregnancy, I'm amazed at how effortless it's been and at how healthy I've been. Maybe Princess Di, and other women her age, have it easier, but I've seen no evidence of my body's falling into pieces." Another woman in her late thirties, pregnant with her second child, sees real advantages to an over-35 pregnancy: "A woman in her late thirties is not usually as vain as a 20-year-old. She's not as bothered by looking different, being less agile, wearing flat shoes. The narcissism of youth has worn away, and she can take the changes in her appearance more in stride."

You may also be more accepting than a younger woman of the changes in your physical condition. You may not even notice temporary discomforts as much. And your body is *not* likely to fall to pieces. Certain conditions that you may already have—such as varicose veins or back ailments—may worsen during pregnancy, but you are no more likely than a younger woman to suffer severely with the other common discomforts of pregnancy. Nor are you more likely to have a rough time getting back into shape after the pregnancy if you were in good physical condition at the start.

For women of any age, pregnancy comes in three stages, with the first and third being filled with most of pregnancy's complaints. In between there are three months in which the morning sickness of the first trimester is mostly a memory, and the swollen feet and fingers a concern of the future. During the second trimester many pregnant women feel better than ever, and look aglow with the joy of dawning motherhood. As one pregnant woman put it, "During the first trimester I felt sluggish and sleepy. But during the second, I just felt all that blood pumping." Pregnancy seems ordered in a way to make it bearable, even the worst of it. Tired or headachy or nauseous in the beginning, there are those middle three months of relief and renewal to look ahead to; awkward or swollen or crampy toward the end, wishing the end would come soon, the impending birth of the baby makes it all seem worthwhile.

Pregnancy is not the same experience for every woman, nor is each pregnancy identical for the same woman. From woman to woman and from time to time, there are aspects that will be different. But there are certain universal changes you should be aware of, and certain discomforts that you should be prepared to deal with. The rest of this chapter will discuss them one by one, with suggestions for coping with the complaints. The better informed you are about what's happening to your body, the better your chances are for looking and feeling good during this most exciting time.

Abdominal Swelling: This is the most obvious sign of pregnancy: your abdomen swells into the predictable proportions of impending motherhood. Some pregnant women look forward to it as visible proof that they're pregnant, but have second thoughts at the loss of their "girlish" figures. The changes actually begin earlier than you might expect. The waistline of a pregnant woman begins to expand within a month or two of conception, as she finds herself searching through her wardrobe for elasticized waists and wrap-around skirts. By twelve weeks, the area above the pubic bone expands, and by twenty weeks, the navel area also protrudes. By that time, most expectant mothers have succumbed and made the inevitable switch to maternity clothes.

A woman's profile during pregnancy is purported to be a telling clue to the baby she is carrying. If she looks big, then it's a big baby; if her abdomen is high and pointed instead of low and rounded, then it's a boy baby. Unfortunately for the odds-makers, none of that holds true. The shape of a pregnant woman's abdomen has nothing to do with the sex of her baby. And her big size says more about her own musculature than about her baby's weight: A woman with weak abdominal muscles carries her baby farther out.

But even for the strong-muscled, the change in shape is dramatic and not always welcome. It can be particularly hard to take for women who have always been slender. A look in the mirror may be enough to make them cry. Even if they are carrying high and only in the front—with sides and back as slim as always—they may feel dumpy. It can be an especially unpleasant shock during a first pregnancy, when a woman has not yet experienced for herself what it's like to regain her figure after such a drastic change.

But there are also pregnant women who take pleasure in the fullness of their bodies—the symbol of their fertility and their future motherhood. And no matter how they seem to others, they seem beautiful to themselves. One recently pregnant woman says that she kept her self-image frozen at the point she found most pleasing: "If I caught a glimpse of myself in the store window during the last six weeks of pregnancy, I wouldn't recognize that big mountain of a woman as me. The image, in my mind, was of how I looked in my middle months, the glow that said I was happy, the maternity clothes that said I was more fashionable than fat. In actuality, I may have looked like hell, but it never registered with me." Even women who accept the reality of their late-pregnancy bodies may find them full of beauty, and bursting with new life.

Backache: Backache is one of the most common complaints of pregnancy, especially common to women who have had back trouble before. That makes women over 35 more at risk because they are more likely than younger women to have such preexisting back problems as pinched nerves, slipped disks, or injuries. Back trouble develops or worsens during pregnancy for several reasons, including a woman's general weight gain, the heaviness of her abdomen, and the relaxation of her pelvic joints. Her posture changes in a way that places extra strain on her lower back muscles.

If you're prone to back problems, you would be wise to take certain precautions during pregnancy: When you lift objects, heavy or light, bend from the knees and not the waist. Be sure that you have adequate back support when you're seated. Some expectant mothers carry small pillows with them to place in the small of their backs when they're sitting. At night, a hard mattress with a board under it can help you wake in the morning without a kink in your back. Sleeping with a pillow under or between your knees will also reduce back strain. Specific back exercises can be helpful, but don't just ask a neighbor what her regimen is. It's best to consult your doctor for an exercise plan tailored to your body and your pregnancy. Some women find maternity girdles—with heavy elastic in the back and below the uterus—helpful in preventing or relieving back problems. If you're careful, by day and by night, pregnancy does not have to mean an aching back.

Bowel Changes: (See also Hemorrhoids, p. 35) Bowel functions go haywire during pregnancy. Many pregnant women suffer from chronic constipation, some are gassy, some experience bowel movements that are looser than usual. Sometimes the prenatal vitamins or iron supplements that are taken change the bowel functions. Pregnancy-related hormones that relax the smooth muscles of the digestive tract may cause irregularity. And the increased pressure of the uterus on the intestines may lead to constipation.

Those are the reasons, but what are the remedies? Constipation is best treated by adding roughage to the diet—eating more fresh fruit, bran, and raw vegetables than usual. (A working woman can munch on some high-fiber snacks at the office, such as a granola bar, a bran muffin, raisins, or other dried fruits.) One pregnant career woman who suffered from "total constipation" kept fruit in her desk and ate it constantly. It did not do as good a job as she would have liked, so she consulted her obstetrician about taking a stool softener. If you find that a change in your diet is not effective in alleviating constipation, a stool softener might be a good idea for you, too, but ask your doctor before you try it. If your problem is loose movements, but you are not going more often than usual, there is nothing that you need do about it. It is a normal, harmless, and temporary change of pregnancy. But if your movements are loose and very frequent, you should let your doctor know about it. Diarrhea during pregnancy may be caused by a virus or by something you have eaten.

Breast Changes: The changes that take place in pregnant women's breasts are dramatic. Some women love the alterations, and couldn't be happier with their new profiles; others can't wait until everything goes back down to size. The most obvious change *is* in size. The breasts begin to get bigger about a month after conception, and have further growth spurts during the pregnancy. They also become firmer as the milk glands begin to develop. The nipples are more sensitive, and become erect more easily. Those changes seem similar to the ones experienced by many women before the onset of each menstrual period, though they are more striking now and have a different purpose—preparation of the breasts for lactation.

But there are additional changes, less familiar ones. There may be some itchiness as the skin covering the breasts stretches. The veins in the breasts enlarge, appearing as bluish streaks; that change is also related to lactation, as a greater blood supply is needed in preparation for milk production. In fact, fluid may begin to ooze out of the nipples by midpregnancy. Later in pregnancy, the fluid changes to a yellowish sticky liquid known as colostrum. (Colostrum nourishes the baby for the first few days after birth.)

Many women are more aware of these changes during a first pregnancy. That's partly because there are more changes to notice. This is the first time the pregnancy hormones are acting on their breasts, the first time their milk ducts are multiplying and glands developing to get ready for manufacturing milk. By a second pregnancy, not all that "groundwork" will have to be laid down again, and fewer changes will have to be made.

Many women find the changes in their breasts absolutely enchanting. Finally, they feel, they *have* breasts, and may enjoy showing off their newly developed cleavage. A mother of four delighted in her blossoming body: "After each pregnancy my breasts were left bigger. It was really only a marginal difference, and I'm probably the only one who noticed it. But it was wonderful, anyway." Other women find the changes anything but wonderful. The increased sensitivity brings them pain, not pleasure, and their husband's touch may no longer be welcome. Women who were large-breasted to begin with may get that weighted-down feeling, and a look they don't like. Said one pregnant woman, who has gone from 36C to 38D in just four months, "For someone like me, this is not a pleasant development. I don't want to be a Dolly Parton look-alike."

Whether you start out your pregnancy big-breasted or on the small side, you're probably going to have to upgrade your bra size a few times during this period. You may find that a more supportive bra than you usually wear is more comfortable for you during pregnancy. If you can't find an appropriate one at your regular lingerie shop, you can find bras designed specially for pregnant women at a maternity shop. Some women who don't normally wear bras feel better wearing one when pregnant.

It used to be thought that the support of a bra during pregnancy would prevent sagging later on. But that's not the case. After pregnancy, the breasts are often less elastic, and softer, from their months of enlargement—whether or not a bra was worn. In most cases, the breasts return to about the same size that they were before the pregnancy, though some women notice that they remain slightly larger or are left a bit smaller.

Faintness and Dizziness: If we believe what we see on the silver screen, a woman who swoons into a faint *must* be pregnant. In reality, there is a connection, though not an infallible one. Pregnant women do tend sometimes to feel faint and dizzy, especially in early and midpregnancy. There are two basic reasons for this. The first involves changes in circulation, including an increased volume of blood, lower blood pressure, and the dilation of small blood vessels. As a result, a quick change in posture, such as bounding out of bed in the morning or rapidly rising from a chair, can bring on a spell of dizziness. To prevent dizziness, get out of bed gradually, and stand up slowly.

Dizziness can also be caused by dramatic shifts in blood sugar levels during pregnancy. It's common for a person who skips lunch, and eats a candy bar instead, to experience lower sugar levels a couple of hours later. But this drop in blood sugar will be *more* acute in a pregnant woman, and more likely to leave her faint. Also, if a pregnant woman skips a meal altogether, she might become dizzy. So eating regular meals and healthy snacks will help you to keep your equilibrium.

Many pregnant women become dizzy in a crowded department store or a hot subway; their systems seem more sensitive to such uncomfortable situations. Staying out of them is one solution. But if you can't avoid crowds and you begin to feel dizzy, remember that actually blacking out and falling to the floor is very unusual. Should you feel faint, instead of standing and worrying about passing out, sit down and lower your head and the feeling will soon pass.

Fatigue: (See also Insomnia, p. 36) The first and third trimesters of pregnancy can be very tiring. There'll be times when exhaustion overcomes you, and there'll be no remedy but rest. You may practically nod off in the middle of a book, a meal, a conversation, and hope that the person you're dining with or talking to is no more insulted than is the book's author. You just can't help it. You're pregnant, and you're tired. The fatigue of early pregnancy is thought to be hormonally caused. The exhaustion during the third trimester has more complex origins; it may be due to insomnia (which is common), a heavy weight to carry around, and the rather awkward way of moving about. But in between those two periods is an oasis of time—the middle trimester—when you may feel more energetic, more vital, more lively than even before pregnancy.

For those times when sleepiness prevails, the best idea is to give in to it when possible and to rest. That's not so easy for a working woman, but it can be done. If there's a couch anywhere in your office, find it, and use it during your lunch period after you eat your bag lunch. If there are any other opportunities for catnaps during the day, take them. One lawyer, the mother of four, recalls how short snoozes in the tax library helped her make it through her days, and her pregnancies. A business executive in her late thirties and early in her first pregnancy tries to keep her energy levels up by foregoing her usual two-and-a-half-mile walk to work, and taking the bus instead. She's surprised at how well this change works, and by how well she feels: "I'm the type of person that generally tires easily. When I heard stories about indefatigable women who go to bed at eight o'clock when they're pregnant, I thought I'd be a basket case. But I don't feel much more tired than usual. I think it's my taking the bus that literally keeps me going."

It's not always easy for busy women to reduce their activities substantially or to cut down on their workloads. But there are ways you can slow down a bit, whether it means having one less social evening out, or sometimes riding instead of walking, or watching the nightly news at ten o'clock instead of at eleven and going to bed earlier than usual. Your tired body is telling you that it needs more rest and more sleep.

If you're not out there punching a time clock or preparing an annual report, but home taking care of a baby or toddler, rest may also seem elusive. Try to nap when your child does, leaving the chores to be performed at another time or by someone else. If at all possible, don't turn down any reliable relief help that comes your way. You're not being selfish when you crawl into bed in the middle of the day and depend on substitute child care. You're simply doing what is dictated by your present condition.

Hair Changes: You may have heard it, but didn't believe it—your pregnancy will not only affect the more "obvious" parts of your body, your abdomen, breasts, and other organs, but also your hair. During most of a woman's life, her hair is at different stages, some of it growing and some of it falling out. So her total amount of hair remains about the same; if there is a gradual diminishment, it is not very noticeable. But during pregnancy, the hair usually all snaps into the same phase—the growth phase—and it looks thicker, fuller, and better than ever. (Unfortunately, this effect is usually temporary. In the period between delivery and a woman's return to ovulation, her hair is all in the breaking-off phase. She's then left with about the same amount of hair as she started out with.)

Women report other kinds of changes, too, some of which they say are long-lasting. One woman noticed that her hair became, and stayed, curlier with her first pregnancy. Another woman reports, with some chagrin, the opposite effect. She is 38, pregnant with her first child, and worried. "I have very curly hair, or at least I did. Usually it's curliest in the summer, and I'm the happiest. But it's hot and humid now and my hair is not that curly. I'm afraid that by Christmas the curl will be gone, and I'll look like a pinhead."

During pregnancy, hair frequently becomes more sensitive to various chemical treatments. It's more likely to become damaged and break off during a permanent wave, for example. If you plan to have a permanent at this time, it would be a good idea to tell your beautician that you're pregnant; that will alert your hair care professional to check your hair a little sooner, and to leave the chemicals on for a shorter time.

Some pregnant women decide to forego completely both permanents and hair dying because they've heard that the chemicals used in those processes are absorbed through the skin. Scientific studies have shown that skin is porous enough to allow the absorption of chemicals, but research has not revealed any damage done by these hair-treatment substances, or any relationship between hair coloring or curling and birth defects. If you're intent on keeping as many foreign chemicals as possible out of your body during your pregnancy, you may decide to settle for a good haircut and forget the curl. But, as we've said, there is no scientific evidence of any harm done to you or your fetus from chemical hair-treatment during pregnancy, and you may reasonably decide to continue with your normal beauty-parlor regimen (with particular attention paid to your pregnancy-sensitized hair, as previously described).

Headaches: (See also Sinus Congestion and Allergy, p. 40) Many women suffer from headaches during the first few months of pregnancy, most often of the "sinus" type. They center in the region right over the eyes, and may worsen if you bend over. One pregnant woman who suffered from them said that half her pregnancy exercise class were similarly afflicted; they talked as much about sinuses as about sit-ups. The cause of these headaches seems to be the sinus congestion so common in pregnancy. Some pregnant women get tension headaches. They feel the pain spreading from the back of the neck into the back of the head. If headaches are bothering you, ask your doctor if it's all right to take acetaminophen to relieve the discomfort.

Fortunately, some pregnant women will suffer from fewer headaches than prior to pregnancy. And women prone to migraine headaches may have either improvement or worsening of their headaches during pregnancy.

Heartburn: This is another of those complaints that are more common during the beginning and end period of pregnancy than in the middle. In early pregnancy, heartburn may be mixed in with nausea, and may be the more annoying of those symptoms. Toward pregnancy's end, it can occur as the uterus pushes the stomach up and even flattens it, causing some of the stomach's juices and gases to move into the esophagus (the tube that runs from the mouth to the stomach). The result is a fiery, burning feeling in the lower chest or in the middle of the abdomen. Heartburn will cure itself within a day or two after the birth, but you can protect yourself during pregnancy by watching what you eat. If you're planning on a six-course dinner at a Szechuan restaurant, you may have to pay afterward with that sizzling sensation. It's better to eat small meals of bland foods than large spicy dinners. The food may not taste as good to you, but it will go down a lot better. One woman, 36 and pregnant for the second time, describes her battle against heartburn: "Since I work, I'm always in a hurry. I'll find myself having a cup of coffee for breakfast, skipping lunch, and then trying to make up for it in one big dinner. But then I want to die. So I've made a real effort to eat smaller meals. I still feel a little uncomfortable, but not nearly as bad." If the discomfort strikes between meals, it may help to put something in your stomach, such as a cracker or some milk. If nothing seems to help, ask your doctor whether you should take antacids. Be sure *not* to treat yourself with sodium bicarbonate. It tends to promote water retention, and may work to elevate your blood pressure.

Hemorrhoids: (See also Bowel Changes, p. 29) Hemorrhoids are enlarged veins in the anal area that plague many pregnant women. Expectant mothers are a prime target for hemorrhoids because of their increased weight, their change in bowel functions (constipation or diarrhea can make hemorrhoids worse), and the pressure of the growing uterus pushing on the veins. The tendency toward developing hemorrhoids, whether in pregnancy or not, increases with age.

To prevent or minimize these painful swellings, it's a good idea to keep to a reasonable weight gain, and to try to avoid bowel problems by following the advice in the relevant section of this chapter. If you do develop hemorrhoids, a sitz bath may help ease the pain. The hemorrhoidal preparations you see advertised may also be somewhat soothing. Some women, free of hemorrhoids throughout the pregnancy, develop them after labor as a result of strenuously pushing the baby out. But by two months after the delivery, hemorrhoids are generally no more troublesome than they were before the pregnancy.

Insomnia: (See also Fatigue, p. 32) Many pregnant women have a hard time getting to sleep and a hard time staying asleep. There are so many reasons for their insomnia, it's almost difficult to believe they get any sleep at all. They worry about the baby's well-being, and about their own ability to be a good mother; there's the kicking of the baby, which often seems the most pronounced just after the lights go out; there's the call of the bladder, which can occur several times during the night; and there's the discomfort of trying to find a comfortable sleeping position, what with big belly and hard breasts. "My breasts are almost solid," says one woman, just four months pregnant. "I'm very uncomfortable at night. It's like sleeping on two large cones. I've tried to find a new sleeping position, but so far it hasn't worked." In some ways, the period of lost sleep can be considered a practice run for after the birth, when your sleep may well be punctuated by many interruptions.

Sleep medication is *not* a good idea during pregnancy. As alternatives, you may find that you fall asleep easier if you avoid caffeine-containing beverages in the evening, get daily exercise, and do something relaxing (such as taking a hot bath or reading in bed) before you go to sleep. But getting up during the night seems almost inevitable, so try to relax with it. And try to remember that as you get older you need less sleep. You're less likely than a younger woman to walk around in a daze during the day as a result of your nighttime wakefulness. So this can be considered one advantage of an over-35 pregnancy.

Leg Cramps: It happens to many a pregnant woman in the last half of pregnancy, in the middle of the night. Suddenly, a muscle in the calf of her leg cramps, and the pain is intense. She may wonder if labor will be so bad. Actually, the comparison is not so far-fetched because both cramps and labor involve muscular contraction. But first things first: What to do about the leg cramps? If they happen to you, there are ways to relieve them. You could try standing up, or massaging the affected area, or flexing your foot. One woman has frequent leg cramps and to ease them does many foot flexes; it's become a habit with her. Often she wakes up in the morning to find herself with a flexed foot. Another possible remedy is to try applying heat to the cramped area. But if the cramping happens often, it may be the symptom of a condition that can be prevented—a relative deficiency of calcium. Most often this occurs when a woman is not drinking enough milk or consuming a sufficient amount of other dairy products; as a result, she is shortchanging herself of calcium, and her body is giving her the nighttime message. But some women who do drink three or four glasses of milk a day experience frequent leg cramps anyway. Whatever your dietary intake of calcium, if you are troubled by leg cramps you should ask your doctor about taking calcium supplementation. Calcium supplements will probably reduce or totally eliminate your leg cramping problem.

A patient of Kathryn's provided dramatic evidence of calcium's effectiveness. She hates pills, especially large ones like the calcium supplements Kathryn prescribed. When Kathryn first recommended calcium to help relieve her leg cramping, she didn't like it, but she went along with the treatment anyway. The cramping did become less severe within a few days, and so did her motivation to take the pills. So she gradually reduced her own dosage. When the cramping returned, she went back on the pills—for awhile. She went on and off the calcium regimen three times before she was finally convinced that the calcium did ease her leg cramps. She never learned to like taking the pills, but she liked the relief they gave her.

Nausea and Vomiting: If anyone tells you that the early morning sickness that can hit you at any time of the day is just psychological, don't believe it. The nausea and vomiting of pregnancy are real, all too real to the three out of four expectant mothers who get that queasy feeling. They are thought to be caused by the increased levels of hormones of early pregnancy and are believed to be worst in women whose livers are especially sensitive to those hormones. The nausea doesn't start right away, but strikes first between the first and second missed periods, and is usually gone by the fourteenth to sixteenth week of pregnancy. It can turn mealtime into a horror, and even just being around food into a stomach-turning experience. As one pregnant woman describes the beginning months, "I often had a general feeling of nausea, especially in the evening. Even if I wasn't going to eat, just planning a meal was very unpleasant. I couldn't stand the smell of the food. The best way to describe the sensation is to use one of my kids' favorite words— I just felt yukky."

What to do about that "yukky" feeling? The medicine that used to be available to deal with morning sickness, Bendectin, has been withdrawn from the market by the manufacturer. But you can help yourself by eating small meals at frequent intervals, skipping spicy foods, and eating only what you like. If you go too long between meals, and your stomach empties out, you may get an uncomfortable acidy feeling. Orange juice may also be too acid for you. It's a good idea to have some crackers or dry toast at your bedside to eat first thing in the morning, and if you're working, to keep crackers or other dry foods at your desk for snacking.

But no matter what you do to prevent it, you may still sometimes feel queasy. The feeling may come upon you at a singularly inconvenient time—during an important business meeting, for instance, or perhaps during an outing with your children. After a while, though, you'll realize what the worst time of the day is for you—whether it's in the morning, as for most women, or perhaps late afternoon, as is also common—and try to work around it. You might try to schedule business conferences at a time of the day when you generally feel well. Or if you have children to care for, you might consider hiring a babysitter for your "bad" times so your children will have you at your best.

Morning sickness is not the most pleasant aspect of pregnancy, but be patient, the period of nausea and vomiting will pass.

Quickening: Quickening, the first feeling of life, is always an exciting moment whether in the first pregnancy or in the fifth. During a first pregnancy, movement is usually first felt during the fifth month. It may feel like a gas bubble, or a twinge, or a pinch. It's easiest to feel movement if you lie down and concentrate on the area of the pregnancy; whatever you feel going on there is most likely the baby moving. In subsequent pregnancies, women generally experience quickening about a month earlier because they know more what they're trying to feel.

The baby's movements become more obvious as the months go on. What's at first just a flutter eventually becomes a full-fledged kick—not a painful one, but a reminder that there's someone in there who won't be in there long. The baby's pushes and pokes may sometimes make your abdomen undulate—an interesting sight for your husband and your other children as well as for you. If you feel a lot of pokes and well-placed kicks, you and your mate may decide that the kicker is sure to be a boy. In reality, there is no known relationship between an unborn baby's activity level and its sex. However, babies who are active outside of the womb often begin that activity prior to birth, and the quiet, calm child may be quiet in utero as well.

All three of Kathryn's children exhibited their personalities well before they were born. Paul was constantly moving, always kicking, making his presence very obvious. He was active then, and he's been active ever since. He learned to walk at nine months and climbed out of his crib at a year and a half. Once he climbed on top of the refrigerator. It should have been obvious from those first kicks that life with Paul would be a lot of fun but not too peaceful. During Kathryn's pregnancy with the twins, there was much more action on her left side than on her right. Her "right-hand" baby was so still, it would sometimes worry her. Based on their in utero behavior, Kathryn's daughters' personalities have not been surprising. Kristin, active inside, has the same physical tendencies as her brother. She's very agile, and walked earlier than her twin. Alison, by contrast, never climbs on anything, never gets dirty, and never destroys the furniture. She sits and smiles and asks a lot of questions. She was quiet before she was born, and she's quiet now.

Once you get used to your own internal dynamo, you may be concerned if and when the pattern of activity changes. Until late in the sixth month of pregnancy, fetal movement may be inconsistent, and before the movements become strong you may not notice any action for long periods of time. Later in the pregnancy, if the movement seems to be reduced or to cease, you should notify your doctor because it could be a sign that your baby is in jeopardy.

Sinus Congestion and Allergy: (See also Headaches, p. 34) Almost all pregnant women suffer from sinus and nasal congestion—the swelling of the mucous membranes of the sinuses and nose. As a result, the woman can't breathe as easily as usual. Even her ears may feel plugged up. Pregnancy may seem like one long cold. But you can help yourself to breathe more freely. If you're feeling congested, it's a good idea to try using a cold-water vaporizer in your room; another no-risk idea is to use saline nose drops. In severe cases, an ear, nose, and throat specialist may drain the sinuses. But most cases are tolerable or can be treated much more simply.

Women who suffer from nasal allergies are likely to suffer more during pregnancy. That's because of their increased sinus sensitivity. And yet they may be hesitant to take the antihistamines that can relieve their symptoms. Like most other drugs, antihistamines have not been conclusively proven to be safe during pregnancy. It's best to do without them if you can, and to try other strategies to alleviate your allergic reactions. If you live in the city, you might forego your yearly vacation to the country where your allergy is likely to be worse. If you live in the country, try to spend as much time as possible indoors in an air-conditioned environment. If your allergies remain severe, no matter what you try short of drugs, ask your obstetrician whether the benefits of medication outweigh the potential risks. As Joan recalls, her own attacks of hay fever were fiercer than ever during both her pregnancies, and she spent most mornings between 5:00 A.M. and 6:00 A.M. dripping and sneezing. But she put up with the discomfort rather than chance the side effects of the medicine.

Kathryn has had several patients who have stopped their allergy shots out of a desire to take absolutely no medication during pregnancy. But if the shots are medically necessary, they should be continued. If you have any questions about this, ask your physician. If you suffer from asthma, continued medication may be manda-

tory. A severe asthma attack could endanger the well-being of
your fetus. But ask your doctor what the safest medication would
be for you at this time.

Skin Changes: (See also Stretch Marks, p. 42) If you're a woman
who enjoys getting a good tan, and tans rather well, you'll be
happy to learn that you can tan even more easily while pregnant.
A pregnant woman's skin reacts differently to the sun, getting
darker sooner. But if you're fair-skinned and freckled, the sun
might not be so friendly. You'll probably burn more readily now,
and get blotchy, and have more freckles than ever. Susan, a patient
of Kathryn's, went on a "last fling" vacation to Florida three months
before her due date. She was pale when she left, and hoped to
come back with an enviable tan. Instead, she came back unenviably
burned and peeling, and told Kathryn that her vacation had been
ruined. Her body had been willing, but her skin just couldn't take
the sun.

The solution for many fair-haired women is to stay out of the
sun as much as possible. Toward the end of pregnancy, that's often
a natural desire, as the search is on for coolness and shade. According to one woman, in the eighth month of a pregnancy due
to end in August, "I would no more sunbathe than climb a building
at this point." But for women who do want to sunbathe, or who
spend a lot of time outdoors, or who are planning a Florida get-
away, it's a good idea to wear a sunscreen, and to build up exposure
as gradually as possible.

But even without the sun's assistance, there is often a building
up of pigmentation on many parts of the skin's surface. Moles and
freckles on the body often become darker, as do the nipples and
the colored area around them (the areola). A thin dark line forms
from the area of the navel down the abdomen—a line that remains
until about six months after the birth. Perhaps most obvious, some
women develop a "mask of pregnancy," also known as chloasma.
This refers to darkened areas on the cheeks and forehead. It's the
same kind of skin reaction that develops in some women who take
birth control pills. If it seems unsightly, makeup can be used to
cover it over.

The reason for the increased pigmentation is thought to be hormonal. One of the early pregnancy hormones is similar to a hormone that acts on melanin-producing pigment close to the skin.

In effect, the pigment is receiving a "false message" from the pregnancy hormone, a message that tells it to make more melanin. All this is perfectly normal, unpreventable, and temporary. The areas of darkness gradually fade after delivery.

Stretch Marks: (See also Skin Changes, p. 41) As your skin stretches to cover your expanding body, you may find that red zigzag lines begin to appear on your breasts and abdomen. Those red markings are known as stretch marks, and develop in some women in the last trimester of pregnancy. The question of who gets them is largely genetically determined. If you ask your mother and sister and other close female relatives whether they have those so-called "badges of motherhood," you'll get a good idea whether you too will be so decorated. Some women already have stretch marks from an adolescent growth spurt or other periods of rapid weight gain; that's an indication that their skin is relatively inelastic, and may well develop more markings during pregnancy.

Creams and ointments that purport to prevent stretch marks are *not* effective in doing what they claim. However, since they do lubricate and moisturize the skin, you may find them to be somewhat soothing. The positive thing to remember is that stretch marks begin to fade after the birth, and within several months become almost, though not entirely, invisible. Also, it's not likely that you will develop more stretch marks in a subsequent pregnancy unless it's a multiple birth or you gain a lot more weight.

Swelling: If you think your shoes are too tight toward the end of pregnancy, you might blame the shoe salesperson for fitting you poorly. Actually, it's your swollen feet, not the fitter's faulty measurement, that's responsible. Swelling of the hands and feet is common in the last month or so of pregnancy; wedding rings seem permanently embedded into fingers, and shoes leave strap marks to last you through the night. What's happening is that extra water is held by the tissues during pregnancy, and then accumulates in the hands and feet. Unless swelling is accompanied by such symptoms as high blood pressure, headaches, and visual disturbances, it is nothing to worry about, and not a sign that you have toxemia (a complication discussed in chapter 6). Don't try to reduce the swelling with diuretics. Instead, elevate your feet when possible, and ask your physician whether you should cut down a bit on your salt intake. Even with those measures, you may have to make an extra trip to the shoe store to buy comfortable shoes in a size larger than usual. That's especially true in the summertime, when heat promotes the swelling. The extra purchase is certainly worth it to alleviate the pain and pinching of too small shoes on too big feet.

Teeth and Gums: If you're counting on putting a tooth under your pillow during this pregnancy, you may find that the tooth fairy will not be coming as planned. Despite what your mother may have told you, you're not going to lose a tooth for every baby. That old saying is simply not true. However, you may find yourself at your dentist's office for another problem—bleeding gums. During pregnancy, it's common to have swollen, baggy gums, a condition that gets worse as the pregnancy progresses. The inflammation of the gums is thought to be caused by the hormonal changes of pregnancy.

Using pregnancy as an excuse to avoid dental work is not a good idea. Routine dental care should continue during pregnancy, though you should be sure to tell your dentist that you're pregnant. During this time, any necessary anesthesia should be local, not general. If X rays are necessary, your abdomen should be properly shielded. Although your gums may bother you, it's generally not necessary or wise to undergo extensive oral surgery during pregnancy. Your gums will shrink by themselves, and the bleeding will stop, after the baby is born.

Urination: One of the trademarks of the pregnant woman is her frequent trips to the bathroom. The need to urinate, and urinate often, increases during pregnancy. It is most intense at the beginning of pregnancy, when the uterus is pressing right on top of the bladder, and toward the end of pregnancy, when the baby's head is pressing on the bladder. In the middle stages, the need varies, but it is almost always greater than it was before pregnancy. One pregnant woman reports that she is usually the "camel" type—she would go once in the morning before work and then once again when she got home. But during pregnancy she is becoming all too familiar with the office restrooms, visiting them about five times a day. In many women the increased need to urinate is most obvious at night, when they find themselves waking up one or more times to go to the bathroom. That can be somewhat alleviated by drinking less fluids before bedtime. Other than that, there's not much to do about your increased need to urinate. It's a perfectly normal part of pregnancy, and will subside when your pregnancy is over. (After the delivery, some women experience a more permanent change in their urinary patterns because of the change in position of the bladder after childbirth.)

Varicose Veins: Enlargement of veins in the legs is a common complaint of pregnancy. Women who suffered with varicose veins even before pregnancy may find them getting worse now, more painful and more tender; women who get through one pregnancy without them might not be so lucky the second time. There are three reasons why varicose veins first appear or worsen during pregnancy. One is that there is an increased volume of blood, meaning more of a load for the veins to handle; they must expand to let the blood through. But the uterus is pressing down, making it even more difficult for the veins in the legs to do their work— the second reason they swell into sometimes unsightly proportions. The increased weight of a pregnant woman also makes the pumping harder, and the veins dilate to move the blood through. Many pregnant women undergo these changes in blood flow without suffering from uncomfortable varicosities. But those who have a genetic predisposition to varicose veins may find that pregnancy means painful legs. They will experience an uncomfortable feeling of pressure and of constant achiness. For this particular complaint, age is also a factor. Older women are more likely to have varicose veins already, and to experience a worsening during pregnancy.

There's nothing you can do about your genes, or your age, but there are some factors you can control. By keeping to a reasonable weight gain, and by elevating your legs when you sit down, you are reducing your chances of developing the condition. If you already have varicose veins, you should ask your doctor to rec- ommend support stockings. If your case is fairly mild, you may be told simply to buy the same type of support stockings you wore before pregnancy, only in a larger size, or to purchase maternity support stockings. (The maternity stockings exert less pressure on the abdomen, but they are more likely to fall down than are regular support stockings.) If your varicose veins are severe, your doctor may fit you for a special heavy elastic stocking. Varicose veins can be one of the literal pains of pregnancy, but they do tend to decrease somewhat after the birth, and in some women to go away almost entirely.

For the most part, the conditions discussed in this chapter will disappear once your pregnancy is over. They are discomforts to be endured temporarily as your body goes about the miraculous work of forming a new life. Of course, it's unlikely that you'll experience *all* of them. But those you do experience can be endured more easily if you focus on the positive aspects of your pregnancy—the glow of your skin, your luxuriant hair, the rumblings of your baby getting ready to be born. After all, in comparison with the joy of bringing a child into the world, what's a little heartburn?

3

Your Growing Baby: The Nine-month Miracle

The transformation of your body, though profound, seems less dramatic in comparison to the transformation of the body growing within you. From little more than a drop of genetic material, in little more than nine months' time, a human being is created with potential for transforming the world around it. As this life force is taking shape, you may wonder exactly what form it is taking at any given moment. Is it too small to be seen, or almost big enough to be born? Has its heart begun to beat yet? How developed are its limbs, its face? Just what kind of life is it, anyway?

From generation to generation, pregnant women have had these thoughts, fantasizing about the baby they are carrying. But with recent technical achievements, and advances in the field of embryology, you can do more than imagine. The following is a journey in pictures and words through the developmental phases of an unborn baby. Babies do not all develop at the same rate, of course, but the information in this chapter can add some reality to your fantasies.

One Month: At four weeks' gestation the embryo is about 6 millimeters (just under 0.25 inch) long. It has a body with a head, a trunk, and a tail. The neural groove, which is the start of the nervous system, has sealed over to form a tube; the top of the tube swells to form a brain, which is developing rapidly at this point. The head and neck comprise a full half of the embryo's length, and the beginnings of the eyes and ears can be discerned. The heart has already begun to beat, blood has already begun to circulate. Arm buds and leg buds are beginning to bulge out. The kidneys have started to form, and a primitive intestinal tube is in place. In this tiny creature, just a month old, the beginnings of almost all the organs can already be recognized. Yet it does not yet look like a baby.

Six Weeks: During the past two weeks, the embryo has taken on a much more human appearance. Development has been progressing very rapidly, with growth of a whole millimeter (0.04 inch) a day. The head end is still the embryo's largest part, and it has begun to straighten up from its bent position. The brain is maturing, the eyes are forming. The nose and cheeks have begun to show under the eyes. What looks like a waxy mouth will actually develop into an outer ear. At this point the arms and legs are still short round stalks, but the arm and leg buds show definite signs of becoming hands and feet. The arms have developed further than the legs, paralleling the general growth pattern of humans, from the top down. The nervous system is continuing to develop. But at this point the embryo has only the beginnings of a skeleton. Despite all its progress toward its human destiny, the six-week-old embryo still has a rather large tail between its legs.

Two Months: At the eight-week mark the embryo officially becomes a fetus, and it looks much more human than it did at six weeks. It has eyes, ears, a nose. It is 4 centimeters (1.6 inches) in length. Bones have begun to develop within the limbs and the trunk, and muscles are developing underneath the skin. Hair will soon appear on the upper lip, the eyebrows, and near the palms and soles. All the organs have been established, even the appendix is formed, and the sexual organs begin to take shape. With its embryonic stage behind it, the fetus is entering a period of growth and of perfection of detail. It is getting bigger—and better—all the time.

Three Months: More than two inches in length, and weighing in at a less than hefty quarter of an ounce, the three-month-old fetus is beginning to assume the proportions of a full-term baby. Its face, finally, is starting to look like a face. Its profile is that of a baby's with a rounded forehead, a little snub nose, and a very definite chin. There is also the first evidence of tooth formation at this time—a series of ten tooth buds of both the upper and lower jaws that will form the baby teeth (which will break through the gums when the baby is about five months old). By now, the fingerprints have started to form, a mark of personal identity that will last for life. The digestive tract has become more specialized, as has the liver, an important site for manufacturing red blood cells; the pancreas is developing insulin-producing cells. Sexual differentiation continues, and by the end of the third month it is possible to distinguish, by close inspection, a boy from a girl. The fetus has reached greater maturity in action as well as in shape. At this stage, it is in almost constant motion as it waves and kicks its arms and legs. It is exercising its limbs—but not yet strongly enough for you to feel it.

Four Months: From now on, there are few new developments, but there are still some refinements to be made. The fetus's skin is thin, red, and wrinkled, but later in pregnancy it will thicken, and a layer of fat will develop that will fill out the wrinkles. Sometime very soon your baby will kick hard enough, or flail its arms strongly enough, to give you a very definite indication of its presence. Quickening has occurred, and a new dimension is added to your pregnancy. Your fetus is experiencing something new, too—the ability to hear. Its ears function as early as the fourth month, and there is evidence that it hears many sounds. It can probably hear the rumblings of your stomach, the sound of your voice, the classical music you're listening to, or the sound track of the video you're watching. If you wish to influence your baby's musical taste, now may be a good time to start.

The Second Half of Pregnancy: At the halfway point—the middle of the fifth month—the fetus is 15 centimeters (6 inches) long; by the end of the month it will be 25 centimeters (10 inches) long, which is about half the length of the newborn baby. Fine hair on the head, the back, and the shoulders is continuing to grow, and fingernails and toenails appear. Oil glands in the skin produce sebum, which combines with cells discharged from the skin to form vernix caseosa. Especially large amounts of vernix are found in such hairy areas as the upper lip, the scalp, and eyebrows. By about seven months, the fetus's physical development is almost complete. From then on, most of the outward changes involve growth in length, weight, and strength. Two months later, the fetus is ready to be born, and you can behold with your own eyes and hold in your own arms the miracle of the nine months—your baby.

DEVELOPMENT OF THE EMBRYO AND FETUS

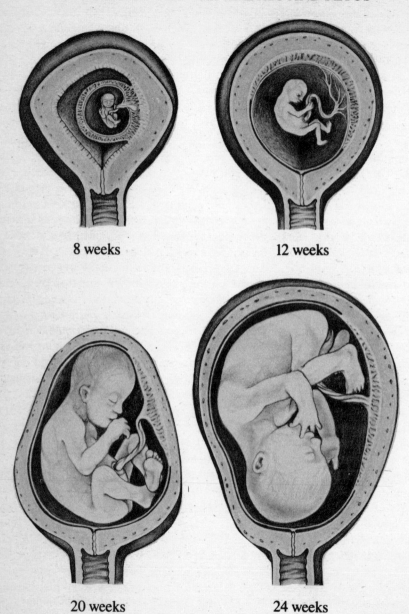

8 weeks

12 weeks

20 weeks

24 weeks

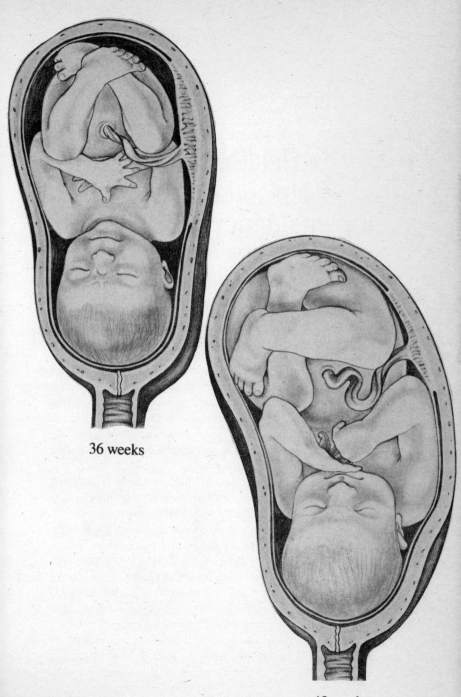

36 weeks

40 weeks

4

Eating for Health: Weight Gain and Nutrition During Pregnancy

For most couples, pregnancy is a time for taking stock of many aspects of their lives. There's often a review of financial resources, living arrangements, family support systems. It is also time to take stock of something more directly relevant to the health of both mother and unborn baby: your dietary habits. You may find that you are not eating as well as you should. It's been estimated that only 20 to 30% of women in the United States begin pregnancy in a good nutritional state. Since pregnancy will place extra demands on you, it's important that you establish healthful eating habits from the outset of your pregnancy.

What's considered healthful now is different than it was just little more than a decade ago. As the medical community has learned more about maternal nutrition and fetal growth, the advice to pregnant women has changed. The main emphasis used to be on severe restriction of weight gain and calorie intake. Very often, the maximum weight gain recommended during pregnancy was just eighteen pounds, with the ideal just ten to fifteen. To go above that, pregnant women were told, was to court a health crisis for both mother and baby. Specifically, a high weight gain was thought to be related to toxemia, a serious complication of late pregnancy (see pages 101–2). If any of your friends or relatives were pregnant in the 1960s or early 1970s, you may remember how little they tried to eat, and how fearful they were of their doctor's admonitions if they tipped the scale too much. Some women would try to ward off the warnings by wearing the lightest clothing possible for weigh-in, and by removing their jewelry—anything for even a few ounces' respite.

But doctors' views have changed since that time. After a decade of intensive research into maternal nutrition, it is now believed that a severely restricted diet is the more dangerous course to follow. Cutting back drastically on nutrients will shortchange the baby in this critical period of its development. Babies born to mothers who have gained too little—fifteen pounds or less—are at a greater risk of being of low birth weight, and of being vulnerable to the associated broad range of health problems. If the mother was underweight to begin with, the risk is accentuated.

Yet another possible risk of undereating has been put forward. When a mother is eating adequately, her daily food intake is used to nourish both her and the fetus. But if she is skimping on calories and nutrients, the baby will draw on the mother's stored fat reserves to meet its nutritional needs. As it happens, fat is a reservoir for substances that may endanger the baby, for example, organic pesticides, toxins, and the trace elements that are in everything we eat. It's possible that even those substances that aren't harmful in normal concentrations may endanger the fetus in the concentrations present in fat. Although that danger is still theoretical, it makes sound scientific sense, and raises further doubts about the sense of the old weight-gain guidelines.

All this doesn't mean that pregnancy should be a feast of fattening foods, that all dietary caution should be abandoned for the pleasures of the palate. It is a time for you to eat sensibly, neither skimping nor overeating, and to form good nutritional habits that can last you a lifetime. It is a time when you are truly eating for two, not in quantity but in quality.

How Much to Gain

Based on current nutritional knowledge, the best weight gain to aim for is in the twenty- to thirty-pound range. For women who were underweight before pregnancy, especially those planning to breast-feed, a weight gain toward the upper end of that scale is desirable. For women who were on the overweight side before becoming pregnant, a weight gain more toward twenty pounds is a better idea. To understand how that recommendation is arrived at, here's a breakdown of just where the weight increase goes. On the average, an increase of about eleven pounds is for the contents of the uterus (including the fetus, placenta, membranes, and the amniotic fluid); the uterus itself gains about two and a half pounds; the breasts weigh, on average, a pound more; and the increased blood volume accounts for another three and a half pounds. To round off the increase, there's another two pounds gained in additional body fluids. So the total increase, simply from being pregnant, is twenty pounds. The extra weight above that twenty-pound figure, which is distributed differently in different women, provides a nutritional reserve for both mother and fetus.

The advantages to the baby of this higher maternal weight gain have been well documented. A substantial weight gain has been linked to higher birth weight and a lower chance of prematurity. And the benefits extend beyond birth. The mother's higher weight gain has been associated with healthier infant growth and performance during the baby's first year of life.

But why shouldn't you try for even a *higher* gain than twenty to thirty pounds, and a more hefty nutritional reserve? Why shouldn't you eat with abandon, adding perhaps forty pounds to your weight, and maybe even fifty? As we mentioned earlier, excessive weight gain does *not* lead to toxemia, nor to any other serious health threat to the baby. In some cases, it may produce a baby too large to be delivered vaginally, and a Cesarean delivery will be required. But that's a rare consequence. What's more to the point is that too much of a gain can make pregnancy quite unpleasant for the mother. Women who put on excessive weight are more likely to get varicose veins, and hemorrhoids, and stretch marks, and back pain. If you think about that as you're reaching for another piece of cake, you might reach for an apple instead. Another thing to think about is what it's going to be like losing that weight after the birth. You may find yourself with an extra twenty or more pounds that you would rather not have, and a wardrobe consisting, for *another* nine months or so, of your maternity clothes. For women over 35, it may be even harder to get that extra weight off—another good reason for not putting it on, and for trying to stick to a twenty- to thirty-pound gain.

Most of the weight should be gained in the latter half of the

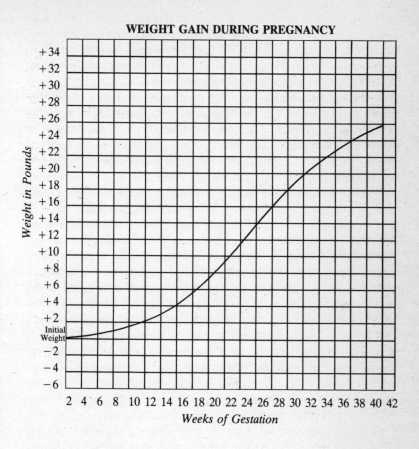

WEIGHT GAIN DURING PREGNANCY

Weeks of Gestation

pregnancy. To get an idea of the appropriate rate of gain through-out the pregnancy, take a look at the chart above. (The chart assumes a total gain of twenty-four pounds. For gains lower or higher, the line would be adjusted accordingly, but the shape of the curve would be about the same.) According to that chart, which reflects current medical thinking, only two or three pounds should be gained in the first three months of pregnancy. Half of the total weight gain—or twelve pounds, in this example—should be reserved for the last three months of pregnancy. The baby is gaining most of its weight at that time, and the mother is most likely experiencing fluid retention.

If your rate of gain is somewhat different than the rate described here, don't be alarmed. There are individual circumstances that can change the curve a bit for some women. For example, some people feel very hungry in early pregnancy, and may exceed the modest recommended weight gain for that period. Or they may be trying to keep food in their stomachs to prevent nausea; as their food stays down, their weight goes up. But others aren't as successful in fighting nausea and vomiting, and find that their weight actually declines in early pregnancy. Your doctor will be keeping a close watch on your weight throughout your pregnancy, and letting you know if a change in food intake is called for.

In some ways, the rate of weight increase is even more important than the recommended total gain. At every stage, the fetus is undergoing critical developmental changes, with brain development occurring most rapidly in the last two months. For a woman who has already gained close to thirty pounds in her first seven months of pregnancy, a starvation diet toward the end is not a good idea. It may adversely affect the infant's birth weight, as well as the baby's central nervous system development. The best idea, if you're in that situation, is to discuss with your obstetrician any adjustments in your diet that might be helpful to you without harming your baby. The recommendation will likely be to slow down your rate of weight gain, but not to stop gaining weight totally, and certainly not to lose weight.

Just how much should you be eating during pregnancy to put on enough weight, at the right time, without overdoing it? There is no single right answer to that question. It depends basically on how much you were accustomed to eating before the pregnancy, and on whether or not you had problems in keeping your weight down. Women who never had to think much about their weight previously probably won't have to struggle with it in pregnancy either. If they just follow their appetites—which generally increase somewhat during pregnancy—they will eat the right amount of food to gain the right amount of weight. Generally, the "right amount" of food means an extra 100 calories a day during the first three months of pregnancy. During the next six months, it means an extra 300 calories daily.

But don't stock up on the grocery goodies yet! That is *not* a lot of extra calories. A tablespoon of margarine, for example, can use up the whole additional 100 calories, as can a single fried egg, or half a cup of rice. As for the extra 300 calories allowable later in pregnancy, eat a hamburger on a bun, or a peanut butter sandwich (sans the jelly), and you've already gone through your fill of additional edibles. That may seem quite all right for women without weight problems, and they may adhere easily to the guidelines, without even having to count calories at all. But for women who never seem to win the "battle of the bulge," pregnancy may seem the perfect time to give up the battle because they're going to bulge anyway. And they may find themselves happily eating all the goodies that they had attempted, with little success, to pass up before. These are the women who may find themselves gaining fifty or sixty pounds during pregnancy, difficult pounds to live with and difficult pounds to lose. These are the women whose appetites may lead them astray.

Joanne was one of those women. When she came into Kathryn's office, she told the doctor that she had gained fifty pounds during her first pregnancy. Ten of those pounds remained with her, and now that she was pregnant again, she wanted to avoid repeating that scenario. Kathryn told Joanne, and her other pregnant patients who have appetite control problems, that they should be on a regimented diet plan for this period, and she recommended such a plan for them to follow. Many physicians suggest following the Weight Watchers program, or similar programs based on well-balanced, common sense diets; other doctors hand out printed sheets of well-balanced low-calorie diet plans. Women who stick to such a diet often find themselves healthier and in better shape after the pregnancy than they were before. (Any such diet should be attempted only under a doctor's supervision.)

Some overweight women, however, undertake dangerous diets during their pregnancy, engendering health risks for them and their babies. These women may view pregnancy as a wonderful weight-reduction opportunity, a time for famine rather than feasting. They know that if they gain little or no weight during this nine-month span, they will lose fifteen pounds or more immediately after delivery. So they eat very sparingly, unwilling to pass up the chance of a seemingly painless loss. But they are playing a dangerous game. Barbara Luke, clinical specialist in maternal nutrition, emphasizes those dangers. As she writes in her book, *Maternal Nutrition*, "This kind of regimen may do irreparable damage to the developing fetus and worsen the medical and nutritional status of the mother."

The fetus may be harmed in various ways by a meager maternal diet. There is the risk of general malnutrition, affecting every area of fetal development. In addition, substances known as ketones may build up in the mother's blood and enter the fetus. It is thought that those byproducts of fat breakdown can do damage to the growing baby. Artificial sweeteners are often used as part of a reducing plan to sweeten coffee or in diet drinks. Because animal studies have raised questions about the safety of such sweeteners, there is some concern about their effects on the developing fetus. It's safer for you to stay away from them during your pregnancy.

Pregnancy is not the time for fad dieting, for eating just grapefruits and eggs, or for an all-protein menu, or for an anything-but-protein regimen, or for mixing up powdered brews instead of eating solid, wholesome food. It is the time to be reasonable and thoughtful about your food intake, and to adhere to a restrictive diet only under the supervision of your doctor.

Over-35 mothers may need to be a bit more careful than other mothers in watching what they eat. Calorie requirements begin to diminish gradually after the age of 30. So the "ideal pregnancy diets" you may come across in general pregnancy books and articles may not be so ideal for you, as they are more likely geared to the higher metabolic rates of younger women. But there is some good news for you "older" women. Older mothers are not the ones most likely to gorge themselves during pregnancy and to gain excessively. According to research studies published in the *American Journal of Obstetrics and Gynecology* and the *British Medical Journal*, the younger pregnant woman tends to gain more weight than her older counterpart. That difference holds true both for first-time mothers and for women who have been pregnant before.

If you are an over-35 mother who is expecting twins, your calorie needs and overall nutritional needs will be greater than if you were carrying just one baby. You should be aiming for a weight gain of about thirty to forty pounds. Even if you gain fifty pounds or so, however, it won't be bad for your babies. It will just mean that you'll have more weight to lose after delivery. But you may find yourself with the opposite problem—instead of worrying about gaining too much, you may be concerned about gaining too little. At times you may even have to force yourself to eat when you really don't feel like it to keep up with the increased nutritional demands of your body and your babies. It's helpful to remember that you are laying down an important foundation for your children's future. Eating somewhat more than you crave is a small price to pay for your babies' good beginnings.

The Food to Eat

Now that you know that you can eat a little bit more than before, you may start figuring out just how to use those few extra calories to their best taste advantage. For the 100 additional daily calories of early pregnancy, you would be able to eat almost a whole piece of chocolate fudge, or four fluffy marshmallows, according to calorie charts (certainly a greater temptation than a fried egg). As for the 300 extra calories a day of middle and late pregnancy, how about a piece of cake smoothed over with chocolate icing, or an eclair, or a couple of ounces of candy? Any of the calorie-rich foods just noted would almost certainly satisfy your very sweetest tooth. However, they are *not* likely to satisfy the nutritional requirements of the growing teeth, and bones, and brain, and other developing organs of your unborn baby. During pregnancy, it is important to get high nutritional value out of the calories you consume. Your needs for protein, minerals, and vitamins have increased, and your diet should be tailored to meet those new needs, even if it means some ho-hum desserts.

To provide you with some guidelines, here is a suggested daily diet for pregnancy:

2 servings of lean meat, chicken, or fish
1 quart of milk (4 glasses whole or skim)
1 egg
1 serving of cottage cheese, or a small extra serving of
    meat, or an extra egg
3 slices whole grain or enriched bread (or 3 rolls)
1 small potato
3 or 4 servings of vegetables, raw and cooked
3 or 4 servings of fruit
3 teaspoons butter or margarine

You can add other foods to your diet, particularly ones with nutritional value, and not the "empty calories" of candy and cookies. You may wish to discuss with your physician a food plan that would meet your individual needs, taking into account your metabolism, your activity level, and your taste preferences. (If you suffer from a medical condition such as diabetes or high blood pressure, your doctor will give you very specific guidelines as to your diet. See chapter 7 for more information on those illnesses.)

To help you stick to a nutritional diet, particularly if you haven't had good nutritional habits before, you might want to know exactly what all those extra nutrients will be used for. The following discussion details the nutrients that should be contained in adequate amounts in your diet, and why they're so important to the two of you you're feeding.

Essential Nutrients

During pregnancy, you should be eating a protein-rich diet. Protein is the most important nutrient during pregnancy because it is vital to the formation and growth of the fetal brain; that organ is more fully developed by birth than is the rest of the infant's body. Protein is also important for the development of other fetal tissue, for the growth of the placenta and the uterus, as well as for the mother's increased blood volume. In pregnancy, the recommended intake of protein is at least seventy-five grams—that's almost a thirty-gram increase over normal recommended levels. Meat, fish, and poultry are excellent sources of protein, as are eggs, cheeses, and milk. A quart of milk contains thirty-two grams of protein, almost half the recommended daily amount. (Milk is an ideal food choice for most pregnant women because it is also rich in calcium and vitamin D.) It's best if the majority of protein you consume is supplied from such animal sources as listed above; they furnish amino acids in optimal combinations.

Pregnant women who are vegetarians must take special care to eat a complete-protein vegetarian diet, not just to eat regular meals minus the meat. They can achieve the proper balance of amino acids by eating dairy products, or from combinations of legumes and grains (such as beans and rice); eat the latter together to get the full nutritional value from these foods. Although it can certainly be done, it requires a great deal of thought and knowledge—as well as iron, and possibly vitamin supplements—to combine vegetarianism with a healthy pregnancy and a well-nourished baby.

Calcium is another nutrient especially important during pregnancy, as it is used for building up the baby's bones and teeth. Pregnant women should consume at least 1200 mg. of calcium a day, a 50% increase over the recommendation for a woman who isn't pregnant. Calcium is a vital part of the diet all through pregnancy, but especially in the last half, when the baby's tooth buds and bones are hardening. If the mother's diet is deficient in calcium the baby will most likely turn out fine, but the mother will suffer the lack. What happens is that some of the calcium from the mother's bones will be slightly demineralized—an effect she probably won't feel at the time, but may well feel later in life. Recent research indicates that such a woman may later be prone to osteoporosis, thinning of the bones, and hip fractures. Drinking a lot of milk when she's sixty or seventy probably won't reverse the process; it's very hard to replace the calcium that was lost from the bones during pregnancy. Better to be sure to drink the milk when it counts the most, before the baby is born.

The best sources of calcium are yogurt, cheese, cottage cheese, ice cream, and, of course, milk. Drinking four cups of milk a day is enough to satisfy the calcium requirement. But some women don't like milk so much, and for others, milk doesn't like them. They are suffering from what's known as lactose intolerance, and experience such symptoms as abdominal cramps, bloating, and diarrhea after they drink a glass of this calcium-rich liquid. For these women, it's wise to consider alternatives—calcium sources that won't be as distressing. Cheese is probably the best choice, and it's versatile enough to be eaten in omelets and sandwiches, with pasta, as a snack with fruit and crackers, or all by itself. Ice cream is another possible substitute, although it is high in calories. It's most appropriate for women who are slim or who have not gained excessively during pregnancy. Some obstetricians prescribe calcium supplements for their pregnant patients who cannot tolerate milk.

Pregnant women have a greatly increased need for iron. Iron is a key component of hemoglobin, the protein in red blood cells that transports oxygen from the lungs to the body cells. During pregnancy, oxygen must also be transported to the cells of the fetus and the placenta, and the fetus must develop its own hemoglobin, which uses additional iron. Few women have large enough iron stores to meet the demands of pregnancy, and it's difficult to get enough iron in the diet without overeating. The result of too little iron may be iron-deficiency anemia, a potentially serious development during pregnancy. It has been associated with maternal illness and death, as well as with premature delivery. But iron-deficiency anemia is not such a common problem today because most obstetricians prescribe iron supplements, starting early in pregnancy and continuing for about a month after delivery. The Food and Nutrition Board of the National Research Council recommends such supplementation. If you balk at taking medication, think about all the liver you won't have to eat just by popping a pill!

A word of warning for women with young children: Keep all iron-containing medications out of their reach. The tablets and capsules can be quite attractive, but also very dangerous to children who swallow a large number of them.

The trend is the same for vitamins as for other nutrients: Pregnant women need more of them. Folic acid, one of the B vitamins, is particularly important, as it is necessary for protein synthesis in the early months of pregnancy. But it is the scarcest vitamin in the human diet. Many pregnant women take it in the form of a vitamin supplement. Other B vitamins—thiamine, riboflavin, and niacin—are also in demand during pregnancy to meet increased energy requirements. The B vitamin pyridoxine is needed for the proper development of the fetal nervous system. The fat-soluble vitamins, A and D, are used for the growth of both maternal and fetal tissues. Vitamin C has an indirect benefit during pregnancy, helping the body to use iron and folic acid.

Although it is possible to eat a diet rich enough in most of these vitamins, it has become common obstetrical practice to prescribe vitamin and mineral supplementation for pregnant women. A daily supplement acts as a kind of safety valve in this era of processed and convenience foods, a time when it's possible to eat a lot and still be nutritionally shortchanged. Scientific evidence now supports supplementation during pregnancy. Studies show that it has a positive effect on the weight of the placenta and the infant, and that it helps to reduce complications during labor and delivery. Women who conceive after long-term oral contraceptive use may have a particular need for supplementation of vitamins C, B_{12}, pyridoxine, and folic acid.

If you've already been taking a vitamin supplement, it's a good idea to bring the bottle, or at least its label, in to your physician to check out what the capsules contain. They may be perfectly acceptable, and you can keep right on taking them throughout your pregnancy. Or your doctor may recommend that you change over to a supplement more appropriate to your current nutritional needs.

What your doctor will *not* find acceptable is the consumption of megadoses of vitamins during pregnancy. Large doses of vitamins A and D can cause hypertension in the mother and birth defects in the fetus. Excessive dosage of the water-soluble vitamins, such as riboflavin, niacin, and thiamine, may adversely affect fetal growth and development. It's become very popular in recent years to take large doses of vitamin C in an attempt to prevent the common cold. It's a controversial practice at any time, but especially during pregnancy. Even if you've found that vitamin C seems to keep you free of colds, better to risk a cold during pregnancy than to chance too much of the vitamin. There was a recent report of a baby who developed scurvy early in life—a disease reflecting a deficiency in vitamin C. A look at the mother's habits during pregnancy revealed that she had been taking large doses of the vitamin. To explain the connection, the scientists speculated that the baby's system had become accustomed to the high level of vitamin C that existed during the pregnancy. But after the birth, there was a sudden deprivation of the vitamin, and the resulting development of scurvy. Although researchers don't know how often that effect occurs, it's that very unknown quality that should make pregnant women wary of taking a lot of vitamin C—or any vitamin—without their physician's consent. It's much wiser to consume vitamin C in the form of citrus fruits and vitamin C-rich vegetables (see nutrient chart on page 62) than in megadoses of vitamin pills.

Liquids

Another aspect of the maternal diet involves how much fluid to drink. It's been said that a pregnant woman should really just eat enough for one, but drink enough for two. Liquids are needed

RECOMMENDED DAILY DIETARY ALLOWANCES
FOR WOMEN
163 CM (64″) TALL AND WEIGHING 55 KG (121 LBS.)

| NUTRIENT | NONPREGNANT | INCREASE | |
		Pregnant	Lactating
Kilocalories	2100	300	500
Protein (g)	44*	30	20
Vitamin A (RE)†	800	200	400
Vitamin D (µg)‡	7.5	5	5
Vitamin E (mg T.E.)§	10	2	3
Ascorbic Acid (mg)	60	20	40
Folacin (mg)‖	0.4	0.4	0.1
Niacin (mg)#	14	2	5
Riboflavin (mg)	1.3	0.3	0.5
Thiamin (mg)	1.1	0.4	0.5
Vitamin B_6 (mg)	2.0	0.6	0.5
Vitamin B_{12} (µg)	3.0	1.0	1.0
Calcium (mg)	800	400	400
Phosphorus (mg)	800	400	400
Iodine (µg)	150	25	50
Iron (mg)	18	Supplement**	0
Magnesium (mg)	300	150	150
Zinc (mg)	15	5	10

* 46 g if under 19 years of age

† 1 µg retinol = 1 retinol equivalent (R.E.)

‡ As cholecalciferol; 100 International Units = 2.5 µg of cholecalciferol

§ T.E. = tocopherol equivalent

‖ Refers to dietary sources ascertained by Lactobacillus casei assay; pteroylglutamic acid may be effective in smaller doses

Includes dietary sources of the vitamin plus 1 mg equivalent for each 60 mg of dietary tryptophan

** Increased requirement cannot be met by ordinary diets; therefore supplementation recommended (see text)

SOURCE: "Recommended Dietary Allowances," 9th rev. ed., 1980. Reproduced with permission of National Academy Press, Washington, D.C.

during pregnancy to help the increased volume of blood to circulate, to aid in the distribution of mineral salts, and to stimulate digestion. Also, a large liquid intake will produce a large volume of urine, and in that way help prevent infections of the urinary tract. By drinking six to eight glasses of beverages a day—not counting milk—you'll be meeting your body's increased need for fluids, and making your pregnancy a healthier experience.

The Question of Salt

If you like to eat pretzels or potato chips with your beverages, you may be wondering if it's OK to continue eating them during your pregnancy, or whether their high salt content might be harmful to you. It used to be thought that too much salt caused the serious complication of toxemia, but that connection has been disproven. In healthy women, salt does not cause any severe problems during pregnancy; only in women with such health conditions as chronic high blood pressure or congestive heart failure should salt intake be very limited. If a woman experiences a lot of swelling toward the end of pregnancy, her obstetrician may advise her to reduce her salt intake somewhat. Following that recommendation may help in relieving the swelling a bit. For most women with uncomplicated pregnancies, it is acceptable to continue eating normal levels of salt. As for the question of pretzels and potato chips, it's not only their salt that may be a problem, but the "empty calories" they provide. It's better to snack on peanuts or raisins with your beverages, and to forego the chips for now, so that you and your baby will get the most out of what you eat.

Healthy Snacks

Speaking of snacks, pregnant women used to be advised to avoid them, and to stick to "three squares" a day. But that's not the best schedule for eating well and feeling good. Many pregnant women begin to feel sick if they eat too much at one sitting. And they may become nauseated, or weak, or dizzy, if they go too long between meals. By eating five or six small meals spaced out during the day, both those problems can be avoided, or at least reduced. But again, even those small meals that are really large snacks should be more chock-full of nutrients than of calories. Peanut butter, cheeses, fruits, beans, raisins, raw vegetables, and yogurt are all nutritious foods that you can eat at home or pack up to take out with you.

Eating Well and Working

Many over-35 pregnant women may find eating well not so easy
to achieve. You may have become used to skipping meals, to eating
a big business lunch and little else, or to working all day and doing
all your eating at night. You've just been too busy to think much
about a balanced diet. But now is the time to change that routine,
and to develop a different, more healthful pattern of eating. Even
if you are working away from home, you can plan for a five- or
six-meal day by packing some snacks to take to the office. Remember to keep them high in nutrients and not so high in calories.
Think in terms of a hard-boiled egg, cheese and crackers, fruit,
raisins, snack-sized yogurt that's available in supermarkets, or a
variety of raw vegetables—not of raiding the office candy machine
for a periodic pick-me-up. You can still go out to business lunches,
but keep them on the light side. You might try ordering, for example, a cold salad or a meat and vegetable platter, or a tuna
salad sandwich. Avoid ordering highly spiced or fried foods. With
so many people dieting these days, you will not feel out of place.
There is no reason why you cannot keep right on going with your
busy career, and at the same time eat in a way that's right for you
now, and maybe even right for you later.

Caution and Controversy

Whether you spend most of your days at the office, or home, or
elsewhere, you may be used to starting them off with coffee, and
to drinking it periodically during the day and into the night. But
now that you're pregnant, should you continue with your coffee
wake-ups, and your coffee breaks? Or could the caffeine contained
in coffee—as well as in tea, in many soft drinks, and in some
therapeutic drugs—somehow endanger your pregnancy and your
baby? This issue is of particular importance to pregnant women
over 35. Apparently, they are more likely to drink a lot of coffee
than are younger women. According to one study of pregnant
women, almost 15% of those over 35 drank four or more cups a
day; that compared to just 5% for the entire population of pregnant
women questioned.

   Animal studies first aroused concern about coffee's possible risks
during pregnancy. That research showed a linkage between caf-

feine and lower birth weight, as well as with skeletal abnormalities in the newborn. In humans, caffeine is known to cross the placenta and to reach the fetus. In the fall of 1980, the United States Food and Drug Administration advised pregnant women to avoid caffeine, or to limit its intake.

Studies that have been conducted in human beings yield conflicting results. Some research indicates that women who drink seven or more cups of coffee a day expose their babies to a higher risk of prematurity. Other research has revealed no link between coffee consumption and the development of congenital defects. In the light of current data, it does not seem harmful for a pregnant woman to drink an occasional cup of coffee. But if you would like to break your coffee habit now, or drink less, you might try some good caffeine-free beverages, such as herbal teas. Or buy some decaffeinated coffee beans that are already ground or can be ground at home. They brew up to a delicious cup of coffee.

Alcohol is known to be harmful to the developing fetus, especially if consumed in large quantities. In 1973, a syndrome was defined that describes the condition of babies born to alcoholic women. This syndrome is marked by growth retardation, mental deficiency, and behavioral abnormalities. Known as the "fetal alcohol syndrome," or FAS, it is usually apparent at birth, as the affected infants have indentifiable facial features and are of low birth weight. Unfortunately, the effects of maternal alcoholism are permanent. The studies that have followed FAS children over time have revealed little improvement. The children continue to be adversely affected in almost every area of their lives, as their motor and mental development remain deficient.

Women who drink heavily during only one part of their pregnancy still expose their babies to risk. Even if the drinking is done only during the first ten or twelve weeks, the baby may be born malformed. There have been reports of women who have gone on one or two "binges" during early pregnancy, having eight or ten drinks at a clip, and then abstained for the rest of the pregnancy. Some of their babies have been born with the fetal alcohol syndrome. A recent study has shown that for women who consume one or two drinks every day during the second trimester, the risk of spontaneous abortions is double that for nondrinkers. Women who drink very heavily the last three months of pregnancy are putting their infants at risk for growth retardation. Alcohol in large doses has been clearly shown to cause birth defects. There is no doubt but that a pregnant woman who drinks heavily is endangering her child. Even if she stops drinking after a few months, or doesn't begin to drink until mid or late pregnancy, the danger is there. There is *no* safe time to drink heavily during pregnancy.

So far, we've been talking mainly about women who drink a lot, and drink often. But how about those who take a drink or two to settle down after work, or have a glass of wine on a special occasion? Are they doing their babies harm? Is even moderate or light drinking a risk not worth taking? The scientific results in this area are not as clear-cut. Some studies have found no increase in abnormalities when the mother's drinking level is less than heavy— under three drinks a day. But other research has found that the babies of these lighter drinkers are affected for the worse by the alcohol intake, particularly in birth weight. Also, decreased Apgar scores (a type of medical evaluation of newborns) have been associated with varying levels of alcohol use.

Such results aren't easy to interpret because of two problems with this type of research. One is that many women tend to make unreliable drinking reports to their obstetricians—either over- or underestimating their alcohol consumption—so that their actual level of drinking is hard to know for sure. Also, women who drink alcohol tend to have other habits that may confuse the results, such as coffee drinking, smoking, or the use of marijuana or other drugs. It's not always easy for researchers to separate out the exact cause of any problems that the babies of these women might have.

The United States Surgeon General recommends that all women totally abstain from drinking while pregnant. Many women do choose not to drink at all during this time. Certainly heavy drinking can have very harmful effects on the baby. There is less known about the effects of light social drinking, but the very lack of knowledge should signal caution. If you feel the need to drink you should ask your doctor about the most recent medical findings. At the time of your discussion there may be newer studies that clarify the question.

Smoking is another habit that is risky in pregnancy, and even moderate smoking can cause harm both to you and your baby. Virtually all complications of pregnancy are increased in women who smoke. Those complications include miscarriages, prematurity, stillbirths, bleeding problems, premature rupture of the membranes, and separation of the placenta, among others. In addition, a mother who smokes is nearly twice as likely as a nonsmoker to deliver a low-birth-weight infant (under 5½ pounds). Some research indicates that there may even be adverse long-term effects for the baby. British investigators looked at 7-year-old children, some whose mothers had smoked during the pregnancy and some whose mothers hadn't. The children of the smokers were shorter in stature, and on average three months behind the other children in their reading skills. Perhaps most unsettling, a study reported on in the late 1970s linked maternal smoking with birth defects.

Many of the negative effects of smoking have been shown to be dose-related. The more cigarettes a woman smokes a day, the less her baby is likely to weigh at birth. The effects are the most serious in women who smoke throughout the pregnancy, and not just during part of it. A recent study of 935 pregnant women in the Baltimore area found that women who either stopped or reduced smoking during their pregnancy gave birth to babies who were significantly heavier and longer than those of women who continued smoking as usual. The best course for you to follow is not to smoke at all during pregnancy. If you can't manage that, even giving up cigarettes for part of the pregnancy would be helpful. Smoking fewer cigarettes a day is another way to lower the risks to your baby. *Any* decrease in your smoking gives your baby a better chance.

Smoking marijuana should be totally avoided during pregnancy for a number of reasons. Its active ingredient is known to cross the placenta, slowing the fetal heart rate and changing fetal brain wave patterns. Some evidence suggests that there is a higher rate of fetal death and birth defects among the offspring of marijuana users. In addition, marijuana smoking presents the same hazards as cigarette smoking, only greater, because marijuana smoke is generally inhaled deeply into the lungs and kept there for as long as possible. Although the hazards of cocaine use during pregnancy have not been studied as intensively, that drug should also be avoided by pregnant women. No high is worth endangering your baby's health or life.

Before you were pregnant, you may not have paid much attention to what you ate, or drank, or smoked. If you were doing anything considered unhealthy, you may have decided that the risk to you, and your body, was well worth the pleasure. But now that you're pregnant there's another body to consider, a developing human being who will suffer the pain of your wrong choices without deriving the pleasure. To protect your baby's future, it's well worth taking the time to think hard about what you eat and drink, and to think long before you smoke. By being cautious now, you can help make your pregnancy safe for you and your baby, and give your child the best possible start in life.

5

Sports and Sex During Pregnancy: How to Enjoy Them Safely

For many women of our generation, "26 Miles" is more than the memory of a song that set us to dreaming about the island of romance so many years ago. It has become also a rallying call for physical fitness, a symbol of something worth aspiring to, the goal of the eighties for women in their thirties. In this age of marathons and other physical challenges, we have found that even as the "over-the-hill" members of the "weaker" sex, we can still keep up, and surge ahead, and achieve feats we never thought were in us. Even in the arena of the bedroom, many of us have found that we are at our peak, and that physically and emotionally, sex has never been so good. We've become aware, as women pushing or past 35, that there is *nothing* we cannot do.

But what about now? What effect will pregnancy have on the sports activities and exercise regimens and sexual pleasures that have made us feel so good about ourselves and proud of our bodies? Will expectant motherhood mean hanging up the tennis racket, mothballing the sweatsuit, spending evenings watching TV? In times past, pregnancy was treated as an illness, and the pregnant woman was pampered and overprotected. It was thought that the less she did, the better, by night as well as by day. Considered not only sickly but asexual, she was supposed to keep her thoughts and deeds pure in preparation for the saintly role of motherhood.

But in these times of greater personal freedom and medical knowledge, as well as national passion for "getting physical," it is generally believed that most pregnant women can go on largely as they had before, though with more moderation and caution. Expectant mothers are now common sights on fields and tracks across the country, keeping in shape the bodies that are taking on more portly shapes of their own. And yet there may still be that nagging thought: Is what I am doing really good for me? Is what I am doing hurting my baby?

Your Changing Body

These concerns are well justified for pregnant women of any age and in any physical condition. Pregnancy *does* cause physical changes that make moderation the guiding principle. Some of the bodily changes are obvious; others you may barely be aware of. One of the apparent ones is the growing size and weight of the uterus and all that's inside it. It's not always so easy to carry that weight around, much less to run with it or ski with it. As the pregnancy progresses, the feeling of awkwardness, of being "weighed down," generally increases. Your growing abdomen has still other effects on your sporting life. It will change your center of gravity, making you more likely to fall or lose your balance. It can also lead to lordosis, better known as swayback, a postural shift that can make you prone to backache. There are other, more subtle changes going on. Two circulating hormones, prolactin and relaxin, loosen and soften the ligaments and joints of the body, making movement more difficult and balance harder to achieve. Also, there is often a softening of the joint between the pubic bones and sometimes even a separation of those bones. So all in all, moving around a lot may give you that "jiggly" feeling.

During pregnancy, the volume of blood in the body increases, and the heart has to work harder to pump it throughout the system. Exercise places even more demands on the heart. The result is that you will tire more easily than you usually do. There may also be another result of exercise, a potentially more serious one, but one that has not yet been scientifically confirmed. That is that strenuous activity will take necessary blood and oxygen away from the growing fetus, redistributing it to the mother's muscles. If that were to happen, and the fetus received an inadequate supply of oxygen, the baby might be born quite small and seemingly malnourished—similar to a baby born to a mother who smoked heavily during her pregnancy. But the relevant research has not come up with clear-cut results. However, if you are well conditioned, and don't exercise to the point of exhaustion, your baby is unlikely to be adversely affected by moderate activity.

If the pregnancy is progressing normally, and the fetus growing well, there is no reason to believe that moderate exercise will affect the baby's growth. However, you should discuss with your doctor your individual situation, and find out if there is any reason for you to lower your activity level. If your baby is growing too slowly, for example, your physician will probably recommend that you spend as much time in bed as possible, lying on your left side. That position seems to increase blood flow to the uterus, and to give the baby the best chance to grow and develop normally.

There are other complications of pregnancy that may make sports and exercise too great a risk. For women who experience bleeding, premature dilation of the cervix, premature contractions, or placenta previa (a low-lying placenta), or who have experienced frequent miscarriages in the past, a thorough discussion with the obstetrician is in order before undertaking any exercise program. In such problem pregnancies, the obstetrician often recommends avoiding exercise completely. In multiple pregnancies, a common problem is delivering too early because of the extra pressure on the cervix; exercise would only increase that pressure and perhaps hasten the births. Another possible problem is inadequate blood flow to each of the fetuses. Exercise might aggravate that condition as well. So it's best for mothers carrying more than one to rest up as much as possible. If you think about what's in store for you once your babies are on the scene, you may not mind taking it easy while you can.

So there are a number of factors that can mean severe restrictions on exercise during pregnancy. However, your age is not one of them. Being 35, or 40, or even 45, is not reason enough for making your frequent trips to the bathroom your most vigorous physical activity. Only if there are the complications just described, or such conditions as high blood pressure or heart disease, is there need for extra restraint or a total cessation of sports and exercise.

Keeping Fit and Physical

If you are pregnant and over 35, you can keep in shape, and have fun doing it through most of your pregnancy, as long as you exercise with care and moderation. This is not to suggest that you should choose this time to start a vigorous athletic program. But if all is well with you and your pregnancy, you can generally continue at the exercise level you're used to, under your doctor's supervision. As your pregnancy progresses, ycu will probably need to moderate your activity. Most sports will cause you no problems, done in moderation, if you have been doing the activity regularly prior to your pregnancy. Swimmers and joggers don't have to stay out of the pool and off the track; bowlers and golfers don't have to take a nine-month hiatus from gutter balls and strikes, shanked shots and holes in one. You can continue to play tennis and volleyball, to sail, to cycle in safe places (away from big-city traffic), and to get into your favorite yoga positions. Even if your abdomen is lightly bumped in the course of an activity, that's usually nothing to worry about. The baby is quite well protected from most blows.

But starting a new sport during pregnancy is generally not a good idea. Training for a new sport can be exhausting, and exhaustion, as noted before, can have unknown effects on the fetus, possibly compromising its blood and oxygen supply. Also, the muscles that are being used for the first time in a long time are apt to become strained—a particularly uncomfortable situation for a pregnant woman who has so many other physical changes to adjust to. And the exercise can serve to increase the back pain she may already have. To make matters worse, the medications that are routinely used to ease the pain and distress of muscle injuries and backache are generally off-limits to pregnant women.

If you had to choose an ideal sport for pregnancy, it would be a "non-weight-bearing" activity, such as swimming. This is preferable to such "weight-bearing" activities as jogging because of the joint looseness and balance changes that accompany pregnancy. Jogging should never be first taken up during pregnancy, and even long-time joggers should consider reducing their mileage and perhaps their pace. One of Kathryn's patients was a nine-miles-a-day jogger, whom Kathryn urged to cut down on the running as her pregnancy progressed. But she said she was addicted to it, and she did her nine miles for the entire nine months. She paid for it, though, developing a hernia and a severe case of varicose veins.

As your pregnancy progresses, and your body changes become accentuated, it would be a good idea for you to switch over to activities that are less stressful on your muscles and your skeletal system—for example, to go from jogging to walking or swimming. Swimming is a fine sport for pregnant women, even women who have not been doing it regularly. But before you start a swimming program, check with your obstetrician. It is best to start out such a program gradually, to build up slowly, and to stop swimming before you feel really exhausted. It is also better, during pregnancy, to swim at a slow, steady pace rather than to race through a few laps as quickly as you can. If, while you're swimming or doing any other exercise, you experience pain in the chest or severe shortness of breath, stop the activity immediately. And if you experience vaginal bleeding or uterine contractions during or in between your workout sessions, let your obstetrician know about it. Once your cervix begins to dilate, which usually happens sometime in the ninth month of pregnancy, your doctor will advise you to stay out of the pool. There is a slight possibility that swimming, after that point, could lead to an infection.

While pregnancy is a time when you can continue to keep physically fit, it is *not* the best time to try to increase your fitness level, to break your running record, to lower your golf handicap, or to raise your bowling average. You simply don't have the stamina or energy reserves you had before you were pregnant, or the same balance and sure-footedness. It's best to stop doing whatever you're doing before you reach the point of exhaustion. Let your body be your guide in this. To avoid exhaustion you might pace yourself slower, or take a break to rest up. It's a good idea to discuss with your doctor how to modify your exercise program. Although scientists are not sure of the effect of maternal exhaustion on the fetus, that very lack of certainty should signal a cautious attitude. Now is the time to play just for the fun of the sport, not for the thrill of victory. And it's the time to pass up a marathon run.

There may come a time in your pregnancy when your body tells you that enough is enough. For Joan, it happened in the middle of the eighth month. She had gone on maternity leave from work relatively early—after just seven months of pregnancy—so that she could enjoy swimming and golfing during the late summer and the early autumn before her October due date. She figured that once the baby was born her time would no longer be her own. So these would be her freedom days, and she would frolic them away on white beaches and green fairways. But after about three weeks of frolicking, her body began to quit on her. Her twenty-lap habit diminished to ten, to five, and then to a dip and a splash. She went from an eighteen-hole round of golf to pitch-and-putt to miniature golf with the local teenagers. But she admits that she learned to enjoy the luxury of relative inactivity, and to relish the final weeks of quietly preparing for the birth of her baby.

There are certain activities that you would best avoid during your entire pregnancy. Horseback riding, deep-sea diving, water-skiing, and karate, for example, involve too great a chance of injury to be worth doing at this time in your life. Many of Kathryn's patients ask whether they can go downhill skiing. She tells them that it won't directly threaten the fetus, but that the risk of a broken bone is not compatible with a pleasant pregnancy (and even an expert skier can be plowed into by a runaway novice). Kathryn reminds them of the X rays, and the medication, and the cast— all common accompaniments to a serious ski injury—and most of them decide to stay off the slopes. The very image of yourself pregnant and limping may be enough to turn you, for this winter only, into more of a "snow bunny" than a ski champ.

Lazy and Loving It

But what if you were *always* more of a "snow bunny" than a ski champ? What if your idea of a great ski weekend was to sit by a cozy fire, good book in one hand and good drink in the other? There's little chance, now, of wanting to spend more time on the slopes and less in the lodge. Pregnancy does not, generally, provide an extra surge of energy. On the contrary, there's a natural tendency during pregnancy to move less, to exercise less, particularly in the advanced stages. But just as the athletes among us worry about the risks of doing too much during pregnancy, some non-athletes worry about the risks of doing too little. With the recent proliferation of "exercise during pregnancy" classes and books, the fear is that not suiting up and stretching will somehow be harmful to both mother and child. Is it necessary to exercise if you just don't feel like it? Will it be detrimental to your baby if you don't?

The answer to both those questions is no. If you're not an especially active woman, and "26 Miles" still reminds you more of romance than of running, there is no compelling reason for you to change your ways on account of your pregnancy. Your baby will not suffer for your relatively sedentary lifestyle, and there is no scientific evidence that you will suffer more than most women during childbirth because of lack of muscular preparation. In fact, you're on much safer ground than are the expectant mothers who decide that this is just the time to start an all-out physical fitness program, and begin participating in all the sports they've only seen on television before. *Those* are the women who can get themselves and their babies into trouble.

Starting Slow

This is not to say that inactivity is necessary. Some pregnant women, perhaps more aware of their bodies now than previously, and aware of the precious life inside, want to firm up a bit and attain a measure of physical fitness. There are definite advantages, both physical and psychological, to a very careful exercise program during pregnancy. It can increase your muscle tone and your strength, improve your flexibility and cardiovascular functioning, and help give you a general feeling of well-being. In short, it can provide the same kinds of benefits that it would if you weren't pregnant.

But as a pregnant woman, you'll have to be a lot more careful in starting a new activity and keeping it to a reasonable level. *Don't* start jogging now, or any other such strenuous activity. If it's an exercise program you're interested in, *don't* rush to your nearest health club and try to conquer every piece of exercise equipment and excel in every exercise class. Those clubs are not geared to the special needs of pregnant women. A much better idea is to enroll, early in your pregnancy, in a program especially designed for the physical condition and needs of expectant mothers. Such courses will start you off gradually, keep you within safe limits, and offer appropriate exercise regimens for any complaints common to pregnant women, such as backaches and weak abdominal muscles. If such a program might appeal to you, ask your obstetrician to recommend one in your area. Your local Y may well offer an "exercise in pregnancy" course at a relatively low cost. It's certainly worth checking into.

Many "preparation for childbirth" courses offer exercises that may be especially helpful in readying you for the labor and delivery process. Pelvic floor exercises, for example, are thought by some childbirth educators to condition the muscles to propel the baby out more easily and gently, and to get back into shape more quickly after the birth. The actual value of such exercises in helping to ease childbirth has not been proven, but since they can't do any harm, it's not a bad idea to do them as part of your preparation.

But what if you're not one for exercising, and would rather take up a sport instead? There, your choices are quite limited. Such activities as tennis and jogging and bowling are not best begun during pregnancy. An ideal alternative, as discussed earlier, is swimming. It does not subject your body to undue risks or your muscles to undue strain. And because it is a "non-weight-bearing" activity, problems of poor balance and awkward movement are not a liability. Even if your bones don't fit together so perfectly, you can still do your laps.

Another good exercise regimen to start during pregnancy is walking, not at the languorous pace of window-shopping, but at a good steady clip. Done regularly, it will keep you in shape without causing you discomfort or harming your baby. And walking can be an exhilarating part of your day, lifting your spirits as well as your level of physical fitness. But again, don't overdo it. Stop before you feel overly tired. If you've walked too far to return home comfortably, take a bus or call for a taxi. This is *not* the time to try breaking records, or to struggle home just to prove that you can make it.

Pregnancy is a time when you can stay active, or become active, or remain happily inactive—whatever suits you, as long as you talk it over with your doctor, learn about any complicating factors, and always keep in mind the valuable cargo you are carrying inside. Whether you are happier being fit or "unfit," walking briskly in the wind or shuffling slowly to the refrigerator, your pregnancy will most likely not get in your way. But if you're one of the "slow shufflers," think of this as just a temporary reprieve, and plan to increase your physical activity after your baby is on the scene. Your baby will want a healthy mother, and regular exercise will increase your stamina and your ability to meet the demands of motherhood.

Sex and Safety

Just as exercise during pregnancy has become a fashionable subject, so has the issue of sex during pregnancy. In previous eras, it was believed that sexual intercourse could hurt the baby. Today, we know how well protected the baby is in the uterus, protected by the amniotic fluid, the membranes, the uterus itself, as well as the bony pelvis. And so it is cushioned, in most cases, from being directly damaged by the act of intercourse. The turnabout in attitudes has been even more dramatic. Now sex during pregnancy is all the rage; pregnant women, bursting with new life, are "supposed" to feel sexier than ever; the parents-to-be, marveling in their mutual creation, are "supposed" to express their joyfulness and feelings of togetherness in erotic embrace. It is perfectly natural to be sexually active during pregnancy, perhaps even more active than before. But if you find that you just don't feel like having sex during your pregnancy, at least not as often as you used to, because you're too tired or preoccupied or just not feeling very sexy, that's perfectly natural, too. And if you still worry about the possibility of sex harming the baby, you are not alone.

Just what *is* the truth about sex in pregnancy? In Kathryn's practice, it is a question that the majority of pregnant women do bring up. In most cases, she assures them that they can go on sexually as they did before. Although there is some controversy, the weight of scientific evidence supports the general safety of sex during an uncomplicated pregnancy. If all is going well, you can continue to have sexual relations up until the time your cervix starts dilating (as mentioned before, that generally occurs during the ninth month, and your doctor wil be checking for it). Once the dilation begins, there's a possibility that bacteria in the vagina will be pushed up during intercourse and cause an infection. A small proportion of doctors believe that the ejaculation can also produce a problem, and so they recommend use of a condom. Although that is not the general belief of the obstetric community, you might want to ask your own doctor about it.

Most expectant parents today are at least intellectually satisfied that the physical act of intercourse will not injure the baby. But with the recent emphasis on female orgasm, they may question the effect of such contractions on the pregnancy. Can a woman's orgasmic contractions somehow trigger labor early, before the baby is ready to be born? It is true that orgasm occurring during pregnancy involves uterine as well as vaginal contractions, but in a normal pregnancy, such contractions will not precipitate labor. Most studies show no connection between sexual relations, with or without orgasm, and premature labor. Interestingly enough, a study published in the *American Journal of Obstetrics and Gynecology* in 1979 actually found that pregnant women who were orgasmic had a *lower* percentage of premature deliveries than did pregnant women who were not orgasmic. You should be aware, however, that the uterine contractions of orgasm may be somewhat uncomfortable for a pregnant woman. That's an issue that should be discussed with your obstetrician, as should any other questions you have about sex during pregnancy. (Incidentally, the act of intercourse itself will probably not be painful now because the vagina is looser and more lubricated during pregnancy.)

If your pregnancy is a complicated one, a thorough discussion with your doctor about the advisability of sex is a must. Certain problems will make sexual relations too great a risk, and your doctor will advise you to curtail sexual activity either temporarily or for the duration of the pregnancy. For example, if you've had a number of previous miscarriages, your physician may recommend abstaining from sex during the first three months of the pregnancy. If you're bleeding, that recommendation may be especially strong. In most cases, sexual activity will not produce a miscarriage unless the pregnancy is quite precarious. (Miscarriages are most often due to faulty early development.) But if a woman who has had previous miscarriages does have sexual relations, and then goes on to suffer another miscarriage, she may blame herself for the loss of the baby. The guilt may be so painful it's worth trying to avoid.

If a woman has placenta previa, the condition prescribed earlier in which the placenta lies in front of the cervix, she should avoid sexual relations during the entire pregnancy. Jarring from the intercourse, or uterine contractions from orgasm, could cause vaginal bleeding. During the middle trimester of pregnancy, a miscarriage may be caused by a condition known as cervical incompetence— the cervix begins to open prematurely, and early loss of the fetus may occur. Surgery can correct that condition, but until that's performed, sexual intercourse should be avoided. Later in the pregnancy, if the membranes rupture prematurely, or if the cervix begins to "ripen" earlier than it should, sexual abstention is also generally recommended. If there is a multiple pregnancy involved, women are often advised to refrain from sex earlier than are other women because of the tendency to premature labor. By the way, a factor that is not a "complicating condition" in this regard is your age. If your pregnancy is going along smoothly, so can your sex life. Kathryn's over-35 patients are most happy to hear about this.

If your doctor does indicate that sex might be a problem for you, whatever your age, you should inquire whether it's the actual physical penetration of sexual intercourse that would be risky, or the uterine contractions of orgasm, or both. In cases where it's intercourse itself that should be avoided, other forms of sexual activity can be continued, perhaps even tried out for the first time. But in instances where it's orgasm that might endanger the pregnancy, then even oral sex and masturbation to the point of orgasm would be off-limits.

One further note of caution: Some pregnant women have died when air has been blown into their vaginas during oral sex, causing fatal air bubbles in their circulation. Such deaths have been reported in women at various stages of pregnancy, and occur within minutes of the sexual act. Any questions about this very serious risk should be addressed to your obstetrician.

Although this section has stressed factors that might limit sexual activity, the majority of pregnant women can continue to enjoy sex throughout most of their pregnancy. No longer do most doctors prescribe arbitrary time periods for abstaining from sex, whether the first trimester of pregnancy or the last month or two. Instead, they advise each woman individually, and do not limit sex more than medically necessary. This general liberalization of attitude is based not only on improved medical knowledge but on a recognition of the importance of sex in pregnancy. During this time of transition and uncertainty in a couple's life, rewarding sexual experiences can help strengthen ties to one another, ties of caring, and respect, and affection. Your feelings of intimacy and tenderness may well be enhanced through sexual expression as you await, in harmony, the birth of the child your love has helped to create. If sexual activity is prohibited for a lengthy time period, it can be quite frustrating for the expectant parents, perhaps leading to marital strain and feelings of isolation. So without sound medical rationale to indicate otherwise, most couples are generally left to carry on, sexually, any way they want.

The Sexual Patterns of Pregnancy

But what if you don't want to, at least not very much, and not very often? Is a lowered libido reason for concern? Does it mean that you're odd, different, missing out on the fun that every *other* expectant couple is having? If you fear that's the case, it's important to remember that many—perhaps even most—expectant couples are going through exactly what you are, and that pregnancy is quite often a time of diminished sexual desire and activity. A number of studies have looked in depth at the sexual aspects of pregnancy. While their results are not all identical, they do support this common pattern of a less active sexual life.

A recent study of pregnant women concluded that the women, on the whole, were less interested in sex, enjoyed it less, and experienced less frequent intercourse and orgasm during pregnancy than they had before.[1] But there were some interesting, illuminating details within that general finding. For one, sexual satisfaction was less likely to decline sharply in those women who were happy about being pregnant, who felt more attractive during late pregnancy than when not pregnant, and who continued experiencing orgasm. Another intriguing result was that sexual desire did not decline month by month during pregnancy in a continuous fashion. Although it did go down in the first trimester, it actually increased during the second, and then declined again in the third. Some other studies show this same pattern: a temporary resurgence of sexual interest in the middle three months of the pregnancy. One of the pioneer studies in this field, a Masters and Johnson report involving 101 pregnant women, revealed a significant second-trimester increase in sexual desire and responsiveness. Many of those women reported having more sexual interest during that period of the pregnancy than before becoming pregnant. But a general finding of *all* these sexuality studies is a sharp decline in libido and sexual activity in the third trimester of pregnancy, particularly in the last month.

But why should this be so? Without the fear of becoming pregnant to inhibit sexual pleasure, why can't sex be better than ever for most expectant couples? The hormonal changes accompanying

1. This study of pregnant women was conducted at the William Beaumont Army Medical Center in El Paso, Texas, and involved 52 pregnant women.

pregnancy may play a role in the general decline of libido, but scientists have not yet clarified exactly what that role is. They do believe, however, that psychological factors are certainly important in explaining the downward trend. Pregnancy is often a time of anxiety and insecurity—reasons enough for a lowered sex drive. In addition, some expectant couples may still have the notion that sex is somehow inappropriate during pregnancy, better left for after the birth, *long* after the birth. For the pregnant woman, there may be the feeling of being unattractive, especially in this society that sees slenderness as sexy. If she doesn't feel positive about her body, she might not be interested in or up to enjoying bodily pleasures. For the mate of the pregnant woman, there may also be the feeling that pregnancy is not conducive to sex, and the pregnant body not conducive to lust. Or he may begin to see his pregnant mate as maternal, and not yet be able to integrate the maternal and the sexual.

Some researchers have looked at this downward sexual trend, trimester by trimester. In one study, it was found that the most common reasons for avoiding or disliking intercourse during the first trimester were fear of harming the fetus, and nausea and vomiting. In the second trimester, there was still the fear of harming the fetus, joined by general difficulty within the marital relationship. In the last trimester, the main reasons given for sexual avoidance were physical awkwardness and loss of interest.

If the sexual interest of the woman and her husband decline together, it is unlikely to produce much conflict. But if one partner feels as amorous as ever and the other apathetic, conflict may result. There is not one set solution for this situation, but different possibilities that will suit the patterns of different couples and their unique ways of communicating. Communication is the key here, as you and your partner should work together to understand each other's feelings and needs and come to an agreement that will satisfy you both. It may involve a different sexual pattern than you have been used to, or different sexual practices. This is a time for understanding and accommodation and, for many couples, experimentation.

As a woman of 35 or over, how will *you* be affected if your sex life goes on the downslide during your pregnancy? Will you be in better or in worse shape than a younger woman experiencing the same lowered libido? You're probably more likely to have established a somewhat set sexual pattern in your relationship—and so more likely to be unhappily aware that the pattern has changed. However, as a more mature, experienced couple, you've probably undergone such "slowdowns" before, for other reasons than child-bearing. And you know that the return of desire, after a period of sexual torpor, is well worth waiting for. In fact, research reported in the *Archives of Sexual Behavior* indicates that women who have been married longer regain their sexual interest sooner after childbirth, and resume sexual activity earlier, than the relative newlyweds. So once again, your age does not work against you, nor against the return of your full sexuality.

Pregnant and Provocative

But these sexuality studies reveal another side to the story of declining sexual interest. In virtually every study done, some of the participants reported having *more* sex during pregnancy than earlier, and finding more fulfillment in it. In the Masters and John-son research, for example, out of six women closely studied for sexual response, two experienced multiple orgasms for the first time during the second trimester of pregnancy. (The other four continued a previous pattern of multiple orgasms.) In a recent survey of 119 British women, there was a sizable proportion who enjoyed sex more during pregnancy than before—that figure varied between 12 and 28% on any one occasion. So not all women are "turned off" by sex during pregnancy, and not all men are "turned off" by their pregnant mates. In fact, some men consider their wives more beautiful than ever now. They find themselves espe-cially entranced by the fullness and fertility of her pregnant body, and all the more amorous as the due date approaches.

Pregnancy does not mean, automatically, either a deadly or a delightful sex life. Sexual responses are as individual during preg-nancy as they are in every period of life. But there does seem to be a clue available as to how an individual couple will react—a clue that was quite apparent in the British study. According to the researchers, "one of the clearest findings was that individuals showed consistent patterns of sexuality during pregnancy and childbirth which reflected their levels of sexuality before they conceived." Those women who had derived little or no pleasure from sex prior to pregnancy were the most likely to refrain from sex during pregnancy. Those who had a satisfying sex life before were more likely to have a satisfying sex life now.

Even when there is less frequent sex, it is often replaced by something else. That something else is physical closeness—the touching, the holding, the cuddling that convey, nonsexually, that loving and caring still exist. Such physical contact seems to be what many pregnant women want the most, perhaps as a partial substitute for sex, perhaps because it just feels so good. This is a wonderful time for you to explore the many ways to give and receive pleasure that don't necessarily culminate in sex. Anything from affectionate play to total body massage can help you and your mate maintain intimacy, and have fun while you're doing it. It is something that comes most naturally to older couples, who have learned over the years to meet each other's needs and to delight in each other's bodies without the obligatory orgasm at the end. They have learned that to "pleasure" each other is the greatest pleasure of all, and that physical joy can be experienced without sexual release.

Some expectant couples may fear that the sex they miss out on now will be forever gone from their marriage, that the excitement is over, that they will settle down into a routine of dull domesticity. But for most couples, sex will become more than just a memory. In fact, report the British investigators, 80% of the women in their study were back to enjoying sex again by a year after childbirth— just about the same proportion that enjoyed it in the first place. And that's not the only good news. By their baby's first birthday, about one out of ten women were having sex more often than they used to, and one out of four were enjoying their sex lives more than before their pregnancy. So now is not the time to discard your sexy negligees, or your mood music, or your waterbed, or anything else that enhances your sexual pleasure. It is the time to realize that your sexual desires and activities may be different when you're pregnant, perhaps less intense than usual, but that you have a lot to look forward to.

6

Complications of Pregnancy: When Things Don't Go Right

When a woman over 35 becomes pregnant, she is sure to hear that her pregnancy may be fraught with difficulties, the labor fraught with danger, and that she is putting her own health in jeopardy in her foolhardy pursuit of premenopausal motherhood. That negative attitude has been around for centuries, originating in the medical community and then echoed by the concerned friends and relatives of "misguided" older pregnant women. It was formalized in 1958, when the Council of the International Federation of Obstetricians and Gynecologists labeled first-time mothers 35 or older as "elderly primipara" who should be treated as high-risk patients.

Just how high *are* the risks for pregnant women in their midthirties or older? Many studies have been done in an attempt to answer that question. Some have indeed found that risks rise significantly with maternal age. In research done on more than 44,000 pregnancies between 1959 and 1966, for example, the babies of the older mothers were more likely to die at or soon after the time of birth than were babies of younger women.[1] A study from Israel, which looked at 494 deliveries between 1965 and 1974, found that mothers over 40 experienced a higher frequency of complications during pregnancy than did younger mothers. Also, their babies were more likely to suffer from congenital malformations, and to die shortly after delivery.

1. The "perinatal mortality rate" progressively increased from 25 per 1000 babies at maternal age 17 to 19 years, to 69 per 1000 babies after maternal age 39.

Sounds grim, but a new report that looked at 104 such studies published between 1917 and the early 1980s found that the risks of late pregnancy have been greatly exaggerated. The researcher, Phyllis Kernoff Manfield, associate professor of nursing at Pennsylvania State University, discovered that the early research was often contradictory, and that only 10% of it followed scientifically sound methodology. But in more thorough research done in recent years, age-related risks practically vanished. In Manfield's research, she determined that only an increase in the number of Down's syndrome babies could statistically be linked to older mothers (an issue that will be discussed in detail in the next chapter).

Birth defects aside, if an older mother starts out her pregnancy healthy, her risk of complications is virtually the same as that of a younger woman. Only if she has such conditions as hypertension (high blood pressure) or diabetes—illnesses that are more common in older age groups—would the risks to her and her baby rise significantly.[2] The findings of the recent research confirm what Kathryn has seen in her own practice over the years—a practice that includes many over-35 women. If they start the pregnancy healthy, their age will not be a hindrance to a healthy childbirth experience. Their years do not work against them.

Not only are scientific studies improving over time; so is obstetrical care. That Israeli study cited earlier found that about 10% of babies born to older mothers in 1965 died. By 1974, none of the babies born to women over 40 died. According to the researchers, "This achievement reflects the significant progress in obstetrics that has been made during these years." Today's older mothers are better educated, too.[3] It seems that a new population

2. In a study investigating the pregnancies of more than 26,000 black women between 1973 and 1978, the infants of the over-35 mothers had a perinatal mortality rate 1.7 times higher than did infants of younger women. However, when women who had hypertension before pregnancy were not counted in, that difference disappeared. The investigators concluded, "Age alone did not appear to be an important obstetric risk factor for healthy women 35 years of age or older."

3. Between 1970 and 1980, the percentage of first-time American mothers aged 35 to 39 who had completed four or more years of college doubled. The National Center for Health Statistics connects that trend to still another trend—a substantial decline in the incidence of low birth weight among infants born to women in their thirties. The decline has been more dramatic in this age group than in any other. The women who were college-educated were much less likely than other women to have low-birth-weight babies.

of women are waiting until their thirties to have their babies—women who are educated, informed, and who seek out competent prenatal care. These women are healthier than their counterparts of fifty years ago. And today's medical specialists are better equipped to handle the complications of pregnancy when they do arise. So most over-35 mothers can enjoy a safe pregnancy and expect to deliver a healthy baby.

Most pregnant women of any age *will* have safe pregnancies and healthy babies, but complications can occur that make the going a little rougher, and the outcome less than ideal. In this chapter, we will discuss many of the more common complications, as well as ones that are not so common but are quite dramatic in their effects. As long as you and your doctor are well aware of these potential complications right from the start, you will be able to take steps to ensure the healthiest pregnancy possible.

Bladder and Kidney Disease: Bladder and kidney infections are common during pregnancy, especially in women who have had past episodes of them. The urinary tract is undergoing extra stress at this time because the ureters dilate a little, and the flow of urine from the kidneys to the bladder is slowed. The enlarged uterus also impedes the urine flow, making the area ripe for infection. By drinking a lot of fluid, a woman will reduce her risks of urinary tract infection, but it may happen anyway, especially if it's happened before. And rare is the woman over 35 who can't recall the burning upon urination that is the calling card of an infected bladder. Other symptoms of such an infection include blood in the urine, and pain. If a woman has had a previous kidney infection, she will recognize the type of back pain that signals another one. A sudden rise in temperature would help to confirm her suspicions.

A pregnant woman with a history of urinary tract infections should let her doctor know about it; her physician may want to do some periodic testing. A woman with the symptoms described above should also inform her doctor. If there is an infection present, there are antibiotics available that are safe to use during pregnancy. Although it is generally desirable for an expectant mother to take as few drugs as possible, this is a situation that requires medication. To let a urinary tract infection go untreated is to put both mother and child at risk. The mother's illness may lead to extensive kidney damage, and may also result in a premature delivery. So it's better to take the medicine and check the infection before serious damage is done.

Diabetes: Before the advent of insulin, diabetes and pregnancy were often a fatal combination.[4] Today, the availability of insulin has made pregnancy less dangerous to both the diabetic mother and the developing fetus, but until very recently, a diabetic pregnancy still often involved many serious complications. Pregnancy is a stress time for diabetes, a time that unmasks the condition in women who didn't know they had it, and increases insulin requirements in long-standing diabetics. It is thought that a variety of hormones secreted by the placenta—human placental lactogen, progesterone, and estrogen—may be responsible for the disease's increasing severity during pregnancy. Diabetes, which is a metabolic disease caused by improper balance between the sugar in the body and insulin, can produce shock or coma in the pregnant mother if it's not properly controlled. And it can affect the infant in numerous ways. Diabetes is associated with stillbirths in the last month of pregnancy; with large, difficult-to-deliver babies; with premature babies (delivered early because of the diabetes), and with babies with low blood sugar and various other chemical imbalances. Even after insulin's introduction, those were common complications of a diabetic pregnancy.

But in the past several years, there have been tremendous medical improvements that have meant less chance of prematurity, more normal birth weights, fewer metabolic difficulties—in short, fewer problems for mother and baby. The fetal mortality rate has come down to just 3 to 5%, and in some perinatal centers to 1 to 3%, which is the national average for all pregnancies. Maternal mortality is currently negligible. Because of better obstetrical management, including carefully regulated insulin administration and fetal monitoring, a diabetic pregnancy today usually results in a healthy mother and a healthy baby. However, there are women with diabetes so severe that a pregnancy would be ill-advised. Any diabetic should have a consultation with her physician or with a physician who is experienced in diabetic pregnancies *before* deciding to become pregnant.

4. A 1909 study reported a maternal mortality rate of 30% for diabetic women and a fetal loss rate of 65%.

To achieve the good results that are now possible, a diabetic pregnancy must be handled with great care and with the mother's constant cooperation. For a pregnant woman over 35, the most common diabetic problem that will potentially face her is known as *gestational diabetes*—diabetes that first develops, or becomes obvious, during pregnancy. It affects 1 to 3% of all pregnancies in the United States, but is most prevalent in women 25 and over and most likely if diabetes runs in a woman's family. To discover the presence of gestational diabetes, many obstetricians now do a blood screening test of all their pregnant patients between the eighteenth and twenty-fifth week of pregnancy. That test can detect milder forms of diabetes than can urine tests. The blood screening involves, for Kathryn's patients, the following procedure: fasting in the morning, coming into the office and having a glucose drink containing fifty grams of glucose, and then having blood taken an hour later. That procedure might vary somewhat from doctor to doctor. If your doctor does not do this test routinely and you are over 35 or have a family history of diabetes, ask if you can have the screening done.

If the blood screening yields abnormal results, the patient is then given a glucose tolerance test. That means, typically, fasting from midnight on, drinking a solution containing one hundred grams of glucose in the doctor's office, and then having blood and urine samples taken over a three- to five-hour period.

When gestational diabetes is discovered, the first treatment tried is generally a special diet. While the particular diet is individualized, depending on a woman's weight, stage of pregnancy, and the severity of her diabetes, it always involves a substitution of complex starches for concentrated sweets. Candies, table sugar, and cookies are out. Generally, a woman is put on a dietary regimen involving three meals and three to four snacks a day. In a typical diet for gestational diabetes, the carbohydrate intake is watched carefully and divided approximately as follows: 10% of the daily carbohydrate allowance is consumed for breakfast; 5% for the midmorning snack; 30% for lunch; 10% for the afternoon snack; 30% for dinner; 5% for the evening snack, and 10% before bed.

If dietary modifications do not completely control the woman's blood sugar, then she should be put on insulin therapy. The therapy is not so much for her as it is for her baby. A level of blood sugar that would be acceptable in a nonpregnant woman might be too high for healthy fetal development. So many pregnant women are being put on insulin who have never been on it before, and may never be on it again.

One of the major decisions to be made in a diabetic pregnancy is when to deliver the baby. If it's delivered too early, there are all the risks involved in a premature birth. If it's delivered too late, it may *really* be too late—there is a danger that the baby may have died in the uterus. It used to be that a set time was chosen for the delivery, and at that time, perhaps thirty-six or thirty-eight weeks into the pregnancy, a Cesarean delivery would be done or labor would be induced. But now there are tests available that help to pinpoint the best time to deliver a particular baby—the time when it is safer for the baby to be outside than inside the uterus. Because many of these tests are quite new, and because they are used not only in diabetic pregnancies but in numerous other pregnancy complications (such as hypertension, inadequate fetal growth, and for an overdue baby), we will describe them in some detail here.

One aspect of the testing is to make sure that the baby is mature enough to survive after delivery and that its lungs are well developed. The traditional way to determine that is through an amniocentesis (a procedure described in great detail in chapter 8). A variety of chemical tests are performed on the amniotic fluid to assess the baby's lung maturity. An added tool for this purpose involves the use of ultrasound (sonography). Through measurement of the fetal head and fetal abdomen visible on the ultrasound image, as well as the length of certain bones, and the determination of the maturity of the placenta, physicians have even more information available to them to judge the desirability of delivery.

The other aspect of the testing is to try to find out whether the fetus is in trouble and may die if not delivered soon. Tests for this purpose are initiated as early as two months before the due date, and then done as infrequently as once a week or as often as once a day. One test that is still done, though it has lost some popularity, involves the measurement of estriol levels in the mother's urine or blood. Estriol is a hormone produced in the interaction of the mother, the placenta, and the fetus. If its levels start to fall, it's an indication that the whole fetal-placental unit may not be functioning well, and doctors may consider early delivery. If its level stays high, it's one sign that all is well, and the pregnancy can proceed.

In many major centers, this biochemical test has been either replaced by biophysical testing or is done in addition to biophysical testing. The two most commonly used biophysical tests each involve fetal monitoring. In the procedure known as the nonstress test, an external fetal monitor is placed on the mother's abdomen; the monitor records the baby's heartbeat and the mother notes when the baby moves. If the baby's heartbeat goes up after the baby moves, that's a sign of fetal well-being. The woman and her doctor can be quite certain that everything is fine, that the baby is not under unusual stress, and that stillbirth is not in the offing. But if the baby's heartbeat doesn't go up after the baby moves, or if its movements are very slight and infrequent, the baby may be in trouble. In that case, the test is generally repeated, or other tests done to check on the baby's condition.

The other popular biophysical test, known as the contraction stress test, was originally done by giving the woman an intravenous solution of Pitocin (also known as oxytocin, it is the same chemical that is used to induce labor). Enough was administered to cause three mild contractions within ten minutes. Doctors would then note the response of the baby's heartbeat to the contractions. If the heartbeat remained the same, it was a sign that the baby was not stressed, and that the pregnancy could continue. But if the heartbeat decreased after the contractions, that was a sign of stress, and the possibility of delivering the baby was considered. Now, in many medical centers, oxytocin administration has been replaced by nipple stimulation. The mother stimulates her own nipples, which causes her body to produce its own oxytocin and her uterus to contract. The response of the baby's heartbeat is then noted, as described above.

This type of testing has been an enormous boon to the diabetic pregnancy. It has reduced the risk of stillbirths because a baby at risk is delivered early into an environment that's healthier for it. And a baby who is not at risk is not routinely delivered weeks before its due date, making it a candidate for respiratory and other disorders. As fetal monitoring has become more widespread (and as tighter glucose control has led to smaller babies), the Cesarean rate of diabetic mothers has begun to fall, though it is still in the 30 to 40% range. Research is being done on additional biophysical tests involving such things as fetal breathing and fetal muscle tone that may be evaluated using ultrasound.

Once a gestational diabetic has gotten through her pregnancy successfully, as most diabetics do now, she may wonder whether her diabetes is here to stay. Most likely, she won't have it for a time after she delivers. But in a subsequent pregnancy she is likely to develop it again. And she may well develop a chronic case later in life. A recent study indicates that 60% of gestational diabetics develop permanent, overt diabetes within sixteen years. Any woman who has had diabetes during pregnancy should be tested for diabetes frequently during her life. Many experts consider pregnancy a "window into the future" for diabetics.

Older mothers are not only more likely than younger ones to develop diabetes during pregnancy; they are also more likely to have *long-standing diabetes* before they conceive. As noted earlier, any woman who has diabetes should be thoroughly evaluated by her physicians before she decides to become pregnant. Even with today's advances, there are diabetics who have the disease so severely that they should not become pregnant. If a diabetic has severe kidney or eye disease, for example, her doctor may tell her that pregnancy would seriously threaten her health. Even if her doctor gives her the go-ahead to become pregnant, other changes may be necessary before she actually starts trying to conceive. Anyone on diabetes pills would be put on insulin instead because oral diabetes medication is associated with an increased risk of birth defects. Anyone on insulin would probably be placed on an increased regimen because tight control of sugar levels is so important during pregnancy.

Valerie is a woman who realized the importance of tight control. For ten years, ever since her diabetes was first diagnosed, she had been taking pills to control her glucose levels. In planning to become pregnant she told Kathryn of her intention to do everything perfectly right—to be a "perfect" diabetic. So she faithfully measured her blood sugar level six times a day (in a procedure described on page 92) and gave herself insulin. In that way she managed to maintain an almost perfect blood sugar level. Her labor and delivery were totally normal and so was her baby. It had none of the chemical imbalances common to babies of diabetics. Valerie's vigilance paid off, and she intends to be just as vigilant when she becomes pregnant again.

Tight control during early pregnancy has special significance. As many of the problems of a diabetic pregnancy have been reduced if not eliminated, one problem has grown in magnitude—birth defects. Ten percent of babies born to diabetic mothers have a congenital abnormality. And such abnormalities account for anywhere from 20 to 50% of the early infant mortality. This is not a problem for gestational diabetics, whose disease doesn't usually flare up until midpregnancy. But it is a serious problem for long-term diabetics whose disease is not being treated adequately. Very tight control from the time of conception on is crucial to avoiding the tragedy of birth defects.

These type of diabetics are treated by both diet and insulin. For them, *when* they eat is almost as important as *what* they eat. It's important that they not skip meals, and that the total calorie intake remain steady from day to day. If they deviate from that pattern, they may suffer a severe insulin reaction. Very exacting insulin administration, as mentioned before, is vital during pregnancy. Often, insulin requirements increase at this time, and a woman who has had just one shot a day may find that she now needs two or three to keep her sugar levels normal. As an aid to tight sugar control, many pregnant diabetic women have glucose reflectance meters in their homes, devices that allow them to make frequent glucose determinations throughout the day. About six to eight times daily, the pregnant woman will prick her finger with a pin and then put the blood on a chemically treated paper strip. Next, she places the strip in the reflectance meter to get a printout of her blood sugar level. She can adjust her insulin intake accordingly. In this way, she becomes a more active participant in her own care, and helps to make her pregnancy a healthier one.

Now in the experimental stages is another device, a small computerized machine that can be hooked into a blood vessel; it constantly measures the diabetic's blood sugar, and gives her the exact amount of insulin she needs. The widespread availability of this machine would mark a dramatic advance not only for pregnant diabetics, but for all diabetic women and men.

Toward the end of her pregnancy, the long-term diabetic would undergo the type of tests described earlier to assure that the baby is delivered at the optimal time. For diabetics who have been in good control throughout the pregnancy, the birth can be approached in confidence. The chances are excellent that the baby will be completely healthy, without the myriad of problems that were once the bane of a diabetic pregnancy. One extra note for diabetic women who plan to nurse. While breast-feeding itself need not be a problem, doctors have observed that diabetics who follow a "demand" nursing schedule, breast-feeding at variable times from day to day, have some difficulty in establishing good control. A more fixed schedule of nursing seems to work better in the maintenance of steady sugar levels.

Fibroids: Fibroids are benign, fleshy growths in the uterus that are very common, especially in the over-35 age group. Although these tumors grow during pregnancy, the vast majority of pregnant women who have them experience absolutely no problems from them; most don't even know they have a fibroid. In rare cases, these growths do complicate the pregnancy. Those located inside the uterus may cause difficulty with implantation, or irritate the uterus, or cause the uterus to be abnormally shaped. A fibroid may also cause the baby to be in an abnormal position, or if the growth is low down, to obstruct the baby's passage out and necessitate a Cesarean delivery. If the fibroid is located on the outer wall of the uterus, however, it will not affect the pregnancy in any way. Just to repeat, fibroids usually do *not* adversely affect pregnancy.

Sometimes, however, a fibroid may cause pain. Because of its rapid growth during pregnancy, its blood supply may become inadequate, causing degeneration, which may result in severe pain and tenderness. This pain, which usually lasts anywhere from two days to two weeks, is severe enough that it may be confused with appendicitis. If you experience this type of pain you should call your doctor immediately. You may be told to stay in bed and to apply ice bags. But if that doesn't help, and the pain persists, you may be hospitalized. While it's unlikely that your fibroid will be surgically removed during this time, you'll be treated in the hospital with fluids and pain medication. After the pregnancy, the fibroid will begin to recede spontaneously.

Some women have had surgery to remove a fibroid before they became pregnant, and wonder how that surgery will affect the pregnancy. If the fibroid was located on the surface of the uterus, it will probably have no effect. But if it was deeply embedded in the uterine wall, the wall may be weakened to the extent that a Cesarean delivery should be seriously considered. If *any* past uterine surgery has been done—whether for a fibroid removal or to repair perforation of the uterus during a dilation and curettage or abortion—a woman should inform her physician and review the possible need for a Cesarean. In cases where prior gynecologic surgery was done not on the uterus, but on the ovaries or fallopian tubes, there is no increased need for Cesarean delivery.

Herpes: Women who have herpes may fear more than social ostracism. They may fear that pregnancy is an option that's closed to them, that any baby born to them would be marked by their condition. Or, once pregnant, they may fear the Cesarean delivery that they believe they're destined for. In actuality, there is absolutely no reason why a woman with herpes shouldn't get pregnant, as long as she's monitored closely and given special tests in the last month of her pregnancy. Nor is she fated for a Cesarean. The odds are that the virus won't be active during the last week or two before her due date, and that she will be able to deliver vaginally.

But there is a possibility that the herpes will be active at that time, and a vaginal delivery would then be too risky to chance. What would happen is that the baby would be exposed to herpes during its passage through the birth canal, and then might develop an overwhelming, possibly fatal herpes infection. Doctors are becoming more attuned to herpes patients; they are giving them special tests toward the end of pregnancy to find out if the herpes is active. If the herpes virus is active in the period immediately preceding a woman's due date, the recommendation would be for a Cesarean delivery. But if there are no lesions at that time and the virus is quiescent, a vaginal birth would not endanger the baby. If you or your partner have ever had herpes in the past, be sure to tell your doctor so that the appropriate tests can be done to safeguard the baby. Some medical centers perform a viral culture to detect the presence of herpes, while others take a PAP smear from either the cervix or from the area where the herpes lesions appear. Both those methods are usually quite accurate in determining whether or not herpes exists.

There is some evidence that a first attack of herpes early in pregnancy may cause spontaneous abortions; a recurrent herpes attack would not have the same effect. Some medical researchers have postulated that an initial herpes attack during the first trimester could cause birth defects (similar to those produced by a maternal bout of German measles). However, this risk has not been proven conclusively. Because herpes is such a common problem, a great deal of research is currently underway investigating its possible effects on fetal development. If this is a concern for you, ask your doctor about the most up-to-date scientific information in this area.

Hypertension: A major age-related disease that complicates pregnancy is high blood pressure. An older mother is more likely to have it than is a younger one, and to have had it for a longer period of time. As hypertension has had more of a chance to do its damage to her vascular system and other organs, she may begin her pregnancy at a serious disadvantage. A hypertensive woman who is planning a pregnancy should discuss her plans with her doctor. If she is on antihypertensive medication, her physician may switch her to another drug, one that is safer to take during pregnancy. Before pregnancy, it's also a good idea to discuss with the doctor just what the risks of pregnancy will be. The chances are excellent that everything will go well, and that mother and baby will come out just fine, but high blood pressure does heighten the possibilities for many types of complications. In studies, it has been associated with an increased risk of maternal mortality and illness, of fetal death, of prematurity, and of intrauterine growth retardation. Typically, the newborn infant of a hypertensive mother is smaller than would be expected from the length of the pregnancy. That's because the blood vessels leading to the uterus may be constricted during pregnancy, causing the baby to get less blood and oxygen than normal.

The complication of pregnancy known as placental abruption is also more common in a woman with high blood pressure. In this condition, the placenta becomes partially detached from the uterus, and a blood clot forms behind it, before the baby is delivered. The resulting bleeding can irritate the uterus. Also, because part of the uterus no longer functions, less blood and oxygen reach the baby. Slight separation could cause the baby to die. If such separation has occurred or seems imminent, the baby may have to be delivered early. Yet another pregnancy complication, toxemia, is a particular risk for women with preexisting hypertension, although toxemia may also develop in women with no history of hypertension at all (more about toxemia on pages 101–2).

In women with severe hypertension, all the risks discussed above would be greater; a woman might decide that they would be *too* great, and elect not to become pregnant. But in women with milder hypertension that is kept under good control with medication, the risks are much less. In fact, the pregnancy most often runs smoothly as long as the blood pressure is kept down. According to recent studies, fetal mortality for women receiving antihypertensive medication throughout pregnancy is no higher than for women with no history of hypertension. Many women with high blood pressure *can* have a safe pregnancy, as long as they are followed closely and given medication when necessary.

The hypertensive pregnant woman will also be given special dietary instructions. A high-protein intake will be part of the appropriate diet for her condition. Calorie recommendations are made on an individual basis, but may be less restrictive than the average diet in pregnancy because of the tendency in hypertension toward low-birth-weight babies. Moderation in the use of salt is generally advised for hypertensive patients.

During pregnancy, the blood pressure of a woman with or without hypertension generally decreases during the first two trimesters, and then returns to its prepregnancy level in the third trimester, or goes even higher. So in cases of hypertension, the third trimester is potentially the most dangerous for both mother and child. As with diabetes, it is sometimes advantageous to deliver the baby early, out of an environment that may do it more harm than good. And as with diabetes, the tests described earlier (see page 92) may be performed to determine whether the baby is under stress, and whether it is mature enough to survive in the outside world.

Malignancy: We don't normally associate pregnancy with something as serious and as frightening as cancer, but as women get older their chances of developing a malignancy increase. Breast cancer, for example, begins to occur with greater frequency in the over-35 age group. It's important to continue breast self-examination during pregnancy, though it may be somewhat more difficult to do because the breasts are fuller and denser at this time. Any lump or abnormality should be reported immediately to your physician. Some women in this age group have already had breast cancer, and may wonder if and when it's all right for them to become pregnant. Such women should thoroughly discuss their condition, and their options, with their doctor before becoming pregnant. Because of the hormonal changes of pregnancy and their possible effects on breast cancer, many physicians would caution against pregnancy after a recent breast cancer. But if the woman has been free of the disease for several years, her doctor may feel that it's safe for her to become pregnant.

Other types of cancer, such as leukemias and lymphomas, may also occur during pregnancy or be part of a woman's medical history. A past history of this type of disease usually does not preclude a safe pregnancy for mother and child, though the issue should certainly be brought to the doctor's attention before the decision to become pregnant is made.

If cancer develops during pregnancy, the chemotherapy, surgery, or radiation used to treat it may put the fetus at risk. Those risks must be taken into account in mapping the treatment plan. In some cases, the baby is delivered early to minimize its exposure to anticancer agents; in others, the pregnancy is terminated because the risks necessary to save the mother are too high for healthy fetal development. These cases are all highly individual, and must be approached on that basis.

There are other conditions that complicate pregnancy that are very specific to the state of pregnancy. In this concluding section of the chapter we'll explore six of them, all of them involving serious or fatal consequences to the fetus. Although the chances are that they won't happen to you, pregnant women of any age should be well informed about what can go wrong. In that way they can be somewhat prepared if a serious complication does occur, and all the more relieved when it doesn't.

Placenta Previa: This is the low implantation of the placenta, partially or totally covering the cervical opening. It occurs in about one of every hundred pregnancies. In the beginning of the pregnancy, there is usually no indication that anything is amiss. But in mid or late pregnancy, when the cervix starts to thin out and dilate, the attachment of the placenta to the uterine lining is disturbed, and bleeding may occur. The bleeding is generally painless and intermittent. For some women, the condition is rather mild, and they can continue to function normally. But for others, the bleeding is profuse, and they may require transfusions and months of bed rest. Any woman who experiences bleeding during pregnancy should report it immediately to her doctor. In all cases of complete placenta previa and in some cases of partial placenta previa, a Cesarean will be the method of delivery. The good news for women who have had placenta previa in one pregnancy is that they will most likely not have it in another.

Previous Abortions: Most women who have had induced abortions in the last decade or so have no trouble in carrying a subsequent pregnancy successfully to term. The recent techniques for abortion have been refined enough, and the instruments are small and flexible enough, to leave the cervix intact and unharmed. But some women, particularly those in the over-35 age group, have had abortions before they were legal, or soon after. At that time, the instruments used to induce an abortion were larger than the type used now, and the cervix was dilated more. Also, there was an increased risk of infections or other complications. So there is a small chance that during a subsequent pregnancy the cervix will dilate prematurely, due to the past abortion. Women who have had past pregnancy terminations should be sure to inform their physicians so that the proper monitoring will be done throughout their pregnancy.

Rh Disease: Until the mid-1960s, Rh disease was a major complication of pregnancy that could potentially affect babies born to as many as one out of every eight couples. Those couples were "Rh-incompatible"—that is, the father was Rh-positive and the mother Rh-negative. (There was no problem when the father was Rh-negative and mother Rh-positive or when both were Rh-negative.) During a first pregnancy there was usually no problem because maternal and fetal blood usually do not mix. But during delivery some of the baby's blood might enter the mother's bloodstream, setting up a dangerous situation for subsequent pregnancies. The mother's blood might be sensitized if the baby's blood was Rh positive; she would develop antibodies against that substance. If her next baby was also Rh-positive, such antibodies could cross the placenta and destroy the fetus's red blood cells. The baby could develop severe anemia and many systemic side effects of the anemia, and could even die as a result. Babies were delivered prematurely or given risky intrauterine transfusions. But Rh disease has been virtually wiped out by a vaccine known as Rh-immune globulin, developed in the 1960s, that prevents the mother from developing antibodies. It is generally administered Rh-negative women within seventy-two hours after delivery of an Rh-positive baby, as well as after every miscarriage or abortion, and after amniocentesis. As a recent added precaution, physicians now give Rh-negative women an injection of Rh-immune globulin between the twenty-eighth and thirty-second week of pregnancy. For women so protected, the chances of developing Rh antibodies are very low. To assure such protection, every Rh-negative woman should be certain to remind her doctor of her blood type, and to mention it again at every relevant procedure, such as amniocentesis, and after a spontaneous or induced abortion.

Some Rh-negative women over 35 may have had babies, or abortions, before the development of Rh-immune globulin. Any Rh antibodies that may have developed would show up in a routine blood test done during pregnancy. If such women find out that they are sensitized, they should be sure that their pregnancy is supervised by a physician experienced in high-risk pregnancies. Such women should be followed closely during pregnancy, and may require amniocentesis, intrauterine transfusion to the baby, or premature delivery. With current diagnostic and treatment capabilities, damage to the baby can often be minimized.

Spontaneous Abortions: They are most often termed "miscarriages," and most often dismissed rather lightly by people who have never had them. But they are serious, disturbing events to any woman who has experienced one, perhaps most disturbing to a woman who has waited a long time to become pregnant and doesn't know how easily she will become pregnant again. An older woman is often hardest hit emotionally, perhaps regretful that she didn't try to become pregnant sooner, wary of the ticking of her biological clock. Even if the pregnancy lasted only two or three months, the baby she was carrying was very real to her, as were her hopes for its future. People may tell her that she's overreacting to the miscarriage, but her loss, and her grief, are very real, and her feeling of devastation perhaps very hard to bear. Some women have more difficulty than others in getting through and past the experience. Terry found it extremely traumatic, and eight months later is still feeling the emotional effects: "When I started staining and cramping I knew it wasn't a good combination of symptoms, but I resisted the idea of a miscarriage. I kept thinking 'This is not happening to me.' Even after I miscarried I couldn't believe it had happened. When it finally hit me, it was a terribly sad time for me. I sat and I cried and tried to figure out what had happened. What have I done to cause this? There was the sense that I had failed in some way." Terry finally put it behind her; at least she thought she did. But then she had a dream. "I had a terrible nightmare that I gave birth, but the baby was stillborn. It was just a horrible dream, and when I woke up I felt depressed and I told my husband about it. Later that day I realized that this was the expected due date for the baby I had miscarried. I thought I had gotten over it, but it's apparently much more on my mind than I allowed myself to believe. I would love to have a baby, but the fear of another miscarriage just terrifies me, so we haven't even tried."

The feelings of sadness and self-doubt are certainly understandable, but pessimism for the future is not quite as warranted. In most cases, spontaneous abortion is a chance event, not one that will likely occur repeatedly in a woman's reproductive life. For any pregnancy the odds are as high as one in five that a miscarriage will occur, usually in the first three months. Most often, it occurs because of faulty early development; most often, there is nothing wrong with the mother or father, there is nothing they have done to cause the miscarriage and nothing they could have done to prevent it, and the woman can go on, subsequently, to have a full-term pregnancy.

The most common symptoms of an impending miscarriage are painful cramps in the lower abdomen, vaginal bleeding, and the passage of blood clots, perhaps with white specks in them or pieces of tissue that look like liver. (If possible, that material should be saved and brought to the doctor in a container.) If any of those symptoms occur—even in the middle of the night—you should call your doctor. You may be seen the next day or, if you're in danger of hemorrhaging, treated that night in a hospital. (Less than 10% of miscarriages involve severe hemorrhaging.) If your condition is in doubt, you may be given a sonogram to judge the viability of the pregnancy.

The treatment of a threatened miscarriage is very individual, depending on the woman's particular condition and the physician's medical evaluation of her. Sometimes, the miscarriage cannot be prevented, and a dilation and curettage (D and C for short) may be conducted in the hospital or in the doctor's office. In many cases the woman miscarries at home, and then is checked by her doctor to see if everything has been expelled. If only part of the tissue has been passed, a D and C would be required. *Every* woman who thinks she has had a miscarriage should be checked. If she is Rh-negative she will need the vaccine Rh-immune globulin, described on p. 99. And her doctor will want to see if she has a condition that might have contributed to the miscarriage. Most doctors don't do any special testing after a single miscarriage because the chances are great that nothing wrong will be found with the mother. One miscarriage is generally considered just bad luck. But after two or more consecutive miscarriages, the doctor may look for chromosomal defects, hormone imbalance, a change in the shape of the uterus, or a rare form of infection. In some cases, treatment is possible to reduce the chances of yet another miscarriage occurring.

Toxemia: Despite the advances of modern medicine, toxemia, or pregnancy-induced hypertension, still remains a potentially serious complication of pregnancy. It is not a special problem of older mothers, except of those who had hypertension before they became pregnant. Toxemia, in fact, can be the most severe in very young mothers. But because it is so potentially dangerous, and can happen in any pregnancy, every pregnant woman should know about it.

Affecting about 7% of expectant mothers in the United States, toxemia generally occurs in the last three months of pregnancy. Its symptoms include high blood pressure, increased weight gain, fluid retention, protein in the urine, and perhaps blurry vision and other visual disturbances. If the disease is severe, there may be painful headaches or stomach discomfort as well. If it progresses and is untreated, it may lead to seizures or stroke or kidney damage in the mother, to placental separation, to death of the baby. Although most cases of toxemia are mild, it can be a life-threatening illness. Medical scientists don't know what causes toxemia, but they have begun to treat it more effectively, and more powerful medications are available to prevent serious damage.

For women with mild cases of toxemia, treatment involves bed rest and possibly antihypertensive drugs. If that doesn't control the disease, the woman is brought into the hospital for more careful monitoring. In more serious cases of toxemia, the mother is hospitalized, put on appropriate medication, and early delivery is considered. There are times when the toxemia is so severe that the mother's life is in immediate danger; medication is then given to stabilize her, and the baby is delivered regardless of its maturity or its chances of survival. Depending on the severity of the toxemia and the stage of pregnancy, the baby may be delivered by Cesarean section or by induction of labor.

If the toxemia has been mild, the baby will recover fairly quickly from any ill effects, and the mother's blood pressure will improve over the next few days to few months. But if the toxemia has been severe, it may take several months for the mother and baby to recover fully. Women who have had toxemia in a first pregnancy have a three-in-four chance of not having it again in future pregnancies. Paradoxically, the more severe the case of toxemia has been, the less likely the woman will suffer with it the next time she's pregnant.

A patient of Kathryn's seemed to be having an uneventful pregnancy until her seventh month, when she was admitted to the hospital with severe headaches, swelling, and elevated blood pressure. At that time the fetus was found to be dead as a result of her illness. Labor was induced. When she became pregnant again she was very nervous. She kept thinking that the same thing would occur, that she would lose another baby. She came into the office frequently for checkups and Kathryn watched her very carefully. But this time her pressure remained stable and the pregnancy went along well. Toxemia did not strike a second time.

Tubal Pregnancy: In a tubal pregnancy, the fertilized egg begins to develop in the fallopian tube between the ovary and the uterus. If allowed to continue, this situation will result in a ruptured tube— a dangerous occurrence for the mother. Unfortunately, it's an occurrence that is becoming more common, though doctors aren't sure why. They think it may be related to the increasing use of intrauterine devices or to the tendency toward a larger number of sex partners; those practices may be associated with low-grade inflammations and, in turn, with tubal pregnancies. At least, that is the current medical theory.

Whatever the reason for such an ill-fated pregnancy, it generally shows itself through one-sided pelvic pain and slight vaginal bleeding. A woman may or may not have even realized she was pregnant when these symptoms occur. A blood pregnancy test will determine if there is a pregnancy. (Often tubal pregnancies produce lower hormone levels than uterine pregnancies, and a urine pregnancy test may be positive or negative. An ultrasound examination will help to determine if it is a uterine pregnancy or not.) If all clues point to a tubal pregnancy, it often can be diagnosed with certainty through a minor surgical procedure. The doctor examines the tubes by inserting an instrument called a laproscope in an incision near the navel. If a tubal pregnancy is discovered, further surgery generally must be performed to remove it. If only minimally damaged, sometimes the tube may be left in place and reconstructed or prepared for future reconstruction. But a badly damaged tube is usually removed to help avoid a recurrence of this unfortunate condition.

If the opposite side is normal, a woman who has had a tubal pregnancy can go on to have a successful uterine pregnancy and a healthy baby. However, because in many cases the predisposing factors have affected both tubes, a woman who has had a previous tubal pregnancy will be at higher risk for developing future tubal pregnancies.

7

Amniocentesis: Reducing the Risk of Birth Defects

It is a decision that most pregnant women under 35 do not confront, but that many an older expectant mother spends weeks, even months, agonizing over. Should you or shouldn't you? Should you let nature take its course, and have the baby you're carrying, no matter what may be wrong with it—or should you take advantage of the medical test known as amniocentesis, a safe and highly accurate procedure that can give you foreknowledge of some common serious birth defects, and some control over your own reproductive life?

It is a decision that should be based on a complete understanding of the procedure's benefits and risks, but instead is all too often laced with misunderstandings and misconceptions. Some women believe that amniocentesis can guarantee them, very early in their pregnancy, that they are carrying a baby who will be "perfect"— perhaps not an Olympic athlete or a Rhodes scholar, but sound of mind and body, nevertheless. Others take a much dimmer view. Not only is amniocentesis a procedure of great pain, they believe, but one that can actually *cause* brain damage and other grievous injury to their unborn baby. And besides, think some pregnant women who have already delivered normal children, why should *I* need such a test? Doesn't one normal baby guarantee another?

Unfortunately, some physicians do little to clarify the issue. Some don't even bring up the procedure to their over-35 patients, perhaps out of their own incomplete knowledge, perhaps out of their antiabortion sentiments. Other doctors make the assumption that all their older patients will have amniocentesis. They don't take the time to explain what it will detect and won't detect, or the minimal risks involved. They simply make the appointment; the patient simply shows up on the appointed day, at the appointed hour, doing what her doctor ordered. As one woman recalls, "It was just automatic with my doctor. It was 'You'll have it. That's it. There's nothing to worry about.' He didn't tell me what it tested for, he didn't take a genetic history or send me to a geneticist. There were no pros or cons discussed. He didn't mention the risks, and I didn't ask."

For a number of years after its development, amniocentesis was not frequently done.

In the late 1970s it was estimated that less than 5% of pregnant women over 35 took advantage of the procedure. That was certainly a much lower figure than its proponents had expected, or hoped for. The reasons for it, they believed, were not only the limited information or the reluctance of some physicians but also the possible dangers. Amniocentesis was a riskier procedure then than it is now, and some women simply would not take the risk. Others, who were resolutely against abortion, reasoned that if they weren't willing to terminate the pregnancy, even if severe defects were found, then why go through with the procedure at all? Sometimes fear, not moral fervor, is at the root of a woman's reluctance. A needle in the arm seems bad enough. A needle in the abdomen is simply too frightening to contemplate. One woman, close to but not quite 35, admitted that this was what put her off: "What stopped me was the idea of something entering my uterus in the middle of the pregnancy. It just seemed unnatural. To put it plainly, I wanted no part of the needle."

But in the 1980s, despite such misgivings, amniocentesis is becoming a much more standard, widely done technique for older pregnant women. A recent study of New York State residents exemplifies the trend. In 1979, an estimated 28.7% of pregnant women aged 35 or over underwent the procedure; in 1980, that figure was up to 35.3%. The rate in New York City was 41%, while the rate in some small counties far from genetic centers was zero. Availability was certainly a factor in the difference, but so was knowledge. Women who are fully informed about amniocentesis are likely to seek the information and the peace of mind that the test most often provides. They see it as a way of cutting the risks of an over-35 pregnancy, of giving them more control over their family's future, and of relieving at least some of the anxiety that plagues every pregnant woman, most of all the older ones. Kathryn advises *all* her pregnant patients who are due to give birth after the age of 35 to undergo the procedure.

The Scientific Story

The facts about amniocentesis are as reassuring as the procedure itself, a procedure that confirms for more than 97% of the women who undergo it that their babies are free of the ailments tested for. The procedure is relatively straightforward: A long, thin needle is inserted through the mother's abdomen into the uterus, and a small amount of the amniotic fluid that surrounds the fetus is drawn off with a syringe. That fluid contains body cells that have been shed by the fetus; those cells are tested for possible abnormalities, and the results are ready in about three to five weeks.

Just what abnormalities *can* be tested for this way—and what abnormalities are most *often* tested for—is something that many people do not understand. Amniocentesis cannot detect everything that can go wrong, nor can it give your baby a seal of good health. But what most over-35 women are most concerned about—the presence of mongolism, scientifically known as Down's syndrome—is within the range of this procedure. Down's syndrome, a disorder producing mental retardation, physical retardation, and health problems, is the result of a chromosomal excess. Instead of the normal twenty-three pairs of chromosomes—those strands of genetic material located in a cell's nucleus—the victims of Down's syndrome have an extra chromosome number 21. In order to detect this extra chromosome, as well as other chromosomal defects, scientists grow the fetal cells derived from amniocentesis in a laboratory using tissue-culture techniques. Then they analyze the cells for abnormalities, including extra and missing chromosomal material. Examples of other problems that can come to light are Patau syndrome and Edwards syndrome. Patau syndrome involves an extra chromosome number 13. Edwards syndrome is produced by an additional chromosome number 18. Both those syndromes involve severe physical defects and mental retardation, and usually lead to death within the first year of life. Though they are much rarer than Down's syndrome, like Down's they increase in frequency with advanced maternal age. Through the technique of amniocentesis and tissue culture, it is now possible to detect every known disease caused by an incorrect number of chromosomes.

There is one other test done frequently on the amniotic fluid withdrawn for study. It is known as an alpha-fetoprotein assay, and it is used to detect defects of the neural tube, the structure in the embryo that later becomes the central nervous system. Two such defects are spina bifida—an opening in the spine that can lead to serious impairment—and anencephaly—the partial or complete absence of the brain and upper part of the skull, a condition that causes the baby to die within a few hours. When a fetus is afflicted with such disorders, there will be an excess of the protein known as alpha-fetoprotein in the amniotic fluid. It serves as a reliable "marker" of the disease, and is routinely looked for because of the simplicity of the test for it and the severity of the disorders it reveals. (This is not done routinely at all centers, however. If you are planning to undergo amniocentesis, ask whether this test will be performed.) The level of alpha-fetoprotein can also be detected through a blood test, and some physicians routinely screen all their pregnant patients for it during the fifteenth to eighteenth week of pregnancy. If the level is found to be abnormally high, then the alpha-fetoprotein level in the amniotic fluid is tested.

For most women over 35, those *without* histories of genetic disease in their families or in their mates' families, those *without* any known chromosomal or metabolic abnormalities in them or in their husbands, those *without* a previous birth where genetic disease was present or suspect, these are the *only* tests done on the amniotic fluid: chromosomal analysis, and possibly alpha-fetoprotein measurement. That certainly leaves a lot of unknowns, but other tests are not performed because they are difficult and time-consuming, and only done for special reasons. With amniocentesis, more than eighty metabolic diseases can be detected, and they are looked for under certain circumstances. For example, if both parents are known carriers of Tay-Sachs disease, an illness most common to Jews of eastern European descent, a certain enzyme would then be measured in the amniotic fluid taken from the mother. Its deficiency would be proof that the child is a Tay-Sachs baby.

But if you are among the vast majority of women who have only the standard tests done, the whole procedure may seem disappointing, almost futile. If so many other things can go wrong, things that won't be detected, why bother? The point you should keep in mind is that chromosomal abnormalities are the most common cause of birth defects, and for every over-35 woman undergoing amniocentesis because of her age, chromosomal analysis is performed. While you won't know *everything* about your baby's health after the test is completed, you will be a lot better informed than it was possible to be just a generation ago.

The Risk Factor

The benefits of amniocentesis seem clear enough—the detection of debilitating, life-shortening disorders, and the possibility of evading them by ending the pregnancy—but what about the risks? What chances are you taking by undergoing the procedure? Would you be exposing your baby to the possibility of brain damage or deformity, the very conditions you would be trying to avoid? You can rest assured that you won't be. The fetus is rarely hit by the needle. The fetus actually tends to move away from the needle. The only evidence of a hit that might be evident at birth would be a little scratch on the baby's skin. Amniocentesis cannot be the cause of heart disease, or a missing leg, or a lower IQ, or anything significant. Nor can it cause a baby to be born somewhat prematurely, say a month or so ahead of schedule. Most problems that might occur from the procedure generally happen within forty-eight hours of its performance, and virtually all within four weeks. There is no need for you to worry about any delayed consequences.

In the rare cases when something does go seriously wrong, it basically means that the baby will be lost. It can happen because infection is introduced into the uterus, or because the amniotic sac ruptures, or because the placenta or umbilical cord is hit by the needle. As a result, either the baby will die immediately, or the uterus will begin to contract and the pregnancy will be lost. Of every 200 women undergoing amniocentesis, studies indicate that 199 will suffer no ill effects, and one will lose her baby. It is important for women who are contemplating amniocentesis to know that there is this risk, albeit a small one. It is also important for her to remember that the chances are 199 in 200 that *nothing* will go wrong.

Amniocentesis has become increasingly safe since its introduction, and even over the last five years. One reason is increasing physician familiarity with it. The more that doctors perform amniocentesis, the more skilled they become at it. And as more women are choosing to undergo it, many physicians perform it on a regular basis, several times a week, or even several times a day. Secondly, there is a growing number of specialized genetic centers where the level of knowledge and expertise gives a couple every reason for confidence. Even within many hospitals, there are units that specialize in this procedure. What was once a procedure exciting for its novelty has become boringly—but reassuringly—routine.

The Age Factor

In this chapter, more than any other, the age of 35 represents a very definite cutoff point. In current medical practice, amniocentesis is not routinely recommended for women under 35 (though they can of course choose to undergo it, and more and more women in their early thirties want the reassurance it provides). But if a woman is due to give birth at age 35 or older, amniocentesis is generally recommended. Why is it more appropriate for older pregnant women? And what makes the age of 35 so special? Why not 34? Or 36? Or 46?

As to the first question, certain chromosomal abnormalities, such as Down's syndrome, increase with increasing maternal age.[1] The statistics regarding maternal age are quite convincing, as a look at the chart on page 110 will show you. For a woman of age 20, for example, the odds of having a baby with a significant chromosomal abnormality is one in 526, studies have shown. At age 30, those odds are up to one in 385. By age 35, the chances have risen again, to one in 179, and at age 40, there is a one in 63 chance of having a baby born with a major chromosomal problem. Those odds, by the way, are no less for a woman who has had one or even a station wagonful of previous children, children glowing with good health. Normal children are absolutely no guarantee against having a future child with a birth defect.

But the question still remains—why 35? Why is that the "chosen" age? In the early years of amniocentesis, the procedure was recommended for women 40 and over. It was performed in younger women only for special purposes, such as detecting fetal age prior

---

1. There is some evidence, though not conclusive, that a father's age has a slight relationship to the incidence of Down's syndrome.

The Age Factor

Maternal Age	Risk of Down's Syndrome	Risk of Any Significant Chromosomal Abnormality
15 or under	1:1000	1:455
16	1:1111	1:476
17	1:1250	1:500
18	1:1429	1:526
19	1:1667	1:556
20	1:1429–1:2000	1:526
21	1:1429–1:2000	1:526
22	1:1250–1:1667	1:500
23	1:1250–1:1667	1:500
24	1:1111–1:1429	1:476
25	1:1111–1:1429	1:476
26	1:1000–1:1429	1:476
27	1:1000–1:1250	1:455
28	1:833–1:1250	1:434
29	1:833–1:1250	1:416
30	1:833–1:1111	1:385
31	1:759–1:1111	1:385
32	1:667–1:909	1:323
33	1:526–1:714	1:285
34	1:417–1:526	1:244
35	1:256–1:400	1:179
36	1:20–1:313	1:149
37	1:156–1:244	1:123
38	1:123–1:192	1:105
39	1:95–1:152	1:81
40	1:73–1:118	1:63
41	1:56–1:93	1:49
42	1:43–1:72	1:39
43	1:33–1:57	1:31
44	1:25–1:44	1:24
45	1:19–1:35	1:18
46	1:15–1:27	1:15
47	1:11–1:21	1:11
48	1:9–1:17	1:9
49	1:6–1:13	1:7

SOURCE: Dr. Ernest B. Hook, "Age and Chromosome Abnormalities," *Obstetrics and Gynecology*, September 1981.

to a scheduled Cesarean delivery, or for gauging the severity of an Rh problem. But as the technique improved, as more physicians became familiar with it, as specialized genetic centers sprang up across the country, the recommended age for prenatal diagnosis began to come down. First, it dropped to 37. That is an age at which there is quite a dramatic increase in the incidence of birth defects. But with the further lowering of risks of the procedure, the recommended age was lowered to 35. A look at the statistics can give you a clearer picture of just why that age was selected. The risk of something going wrong because of the amniocentesis, as mentioned earlier, is 1 in 200 (or ½ of 1%). If you look again at the chart on page 110, you'll see that 35 is the age at which the risk of a serious chromosomal abnormality first exceeds that 1 in 200 figure. Specifically, the odds of having a child so afflicted are 1 in 179. So that is the first age at which the potential benefits of amniocentesis outweigh the possible risks. If the risks are lowered even further in the future, it is possible that even younger women will be urged to have the procedure. But it is unlikely that the test will be made so safe that all pregnant women are advised to undergo it.

At the present time, more than 80% of the women who do have amniocentesis performed are in the age group of 35 and older. For each year over 35, its importance grows, as the likelihood of Down's syndrome and certain other chromosomal abnormalities continues to increase. Exactly why the incidence of these abnormalities increases with age is not known for sure. Apparently the sorting process, which determines the appropriate division of chromosomes between eggs, is more likely to go awry as the egg ages. It may be that the egg has been made more vulnerable by all it has been exposed to—such as radiation and toxins—over time. And a 40-year-old egg has been exposed to more than a 20-year-old egg.[2]

2. Those women who are the most obvious candidates for amniocentesis—those over 40—are *not* the likeliest to undergo it. The New York State study that showed a growing usage of amniocentesis from 1979 to 1980 also showed that women over 40 use it less than do women between 35 and 40. And yet the over-40 women are those who would benefit from it the most. The authors of the study, Dr. Ernest Hook and Dina Schreinemachers, speculate that perhaps those older women are more likely to be strongly antiabortion, even if serious birth defects are involved. Perhaps, also, since many over-40 women already have children, children who are normal, these mothers may mistakenly believe that their families are immune from the specter of hereditary disease.

Seeing With Sound

One encouraging addition to the amniocentesis procedure has been the introduction of ultrasound scanning. On page 89, we described just what ultrasound is, and how it is employed during pregnancy. When used just prior to the drawing of amniotic fluid, it provides valuable information to the physician. For one, by allowing the doctor to measure the head of the fetus, it enables the physician to know whether the woman is far enough along in the pregnancy for the amniocentesis to be done. The ideal time to perform amniocentesis is sixteen weeks from the first day of the mother's last menstrual period. Before that, there may not be sufficient amniotic fluid, and the risk of complications would be higher. The sonogram also confirms that the fetus is still alive—and reveals whether there is more than one fetus in the picture. In addition, it shows the physician just where the pockets of amniotic fluid are, so he or she knows where to aim. And it shows the doctor just where the fetus, the placenta, and the umbilical cord are, so he or she knows where *not* to aim.

The use of sonograms prior to amniocentesis is becoming more and more standard procedure. This modern method of seeing with sound reduces the likelihood of blood mixing in with the extracted amniotic fluid, of a second or third needle insertion being necessary, and of later complications. In some centers, sonograms are being used during amniocentesis as well, to "look" at the needle going in. The recording of images occurs at the same time as the procedure, so the physician knows the exact position of the fetus at every moment, and the position of the needle in relation to the other structures of the amniotic sac. One woman was mesmerized by watching the "action"—not the action on her abdomen, but the action on the screen. "I kept looking up at the screen. I saw a fine line on it moving as the needle was inserted. I just stared. I was absolutely transfixed by what was up there. I was actually seeing the amniocentesis being done from the inside. I was actually seeing my baby move. I kept trying to get it in my mind that this moving image is a living thing. Before that, pregnancy to me was just something that made me vomit. Now I could begin to connect it up with a real live being."

Even women who have the more standard sonogram done—prior to the amniocentesis but not during it—often find it thrilling to see the outlines of the baby. It's an extra added benefit of the procedure, one that highlights the real purpose of the pregnancy—to create a new life. Some mothers and fathers can identify some of the baby's parts, and may be thrilled that they get the right count of arms and legs. For others, what they see seems kind of like an abstract image—one woman said that it looked to her like a giant ear—but it's an exciting sight, nonetheless. In some centers, the parents are provided with an instant photograph of the ultrasonic image to take home with them. Often, it is the very first memento that they tape, ever so carefully and lovingly, into their new baby's baby book.

Where to Go, What to Ask

As we've been discussing, amniocentesis is considerably less risky now than a decade or even a few years back, but you can minimize the risks even further by having it done at the right place, by the right person. If you and your spouse make some inquiries before it's done, you are less likely to have reason for regret after the fact. One of the first steps that you should take is to seek out genetic counseling. Some obstetricians do it themselves, but you may be referred instead to a special counselor with training in genetics. At the counseling session, a detailed medical, pregnancy, and family history will be taken. That will tell the counselor—and you—whether there are any risks present besides that of advanced maternal age. If there are, tests in addition to the standard chromosomal ones may be suggested for you. But even if there aren't, there will be a thorough discussion of the procedure of amniocentesis, its purposes, its hazards, and its occasional failures. (In a small percentage, the cells don't grow properly, and the amniocentesis has to be redone.) You and your husband will be told specifically what your risk is of having a Down's baby, based upon your age. Once you are fully informed, the choice will be left to you whether to go ahead and have the amniocentesis at the appropriate time, or to take your chances without it.

If you decide to undergo the procedure, you should seek out the best possible medical environment for it. Amniocentesis is *not* best performed as an office procedure, by a doctor who approaches it as a once-a-month novelty, with laboratory facilities half a continent away. It is ideally done in a special genetic center, or in a large university hospital, where it has become an accepted routine. Under such circumstances, the rate of complications is lower than that half of one percent that is the national average. (In case your own doctor doesn't refer you to such a center, see the end of this chapter for referral information.) The physician who performs the amniocentesis should be highly experienced and expert at the procedure, which means having more than a once-a-month track record. Ideally, he or she will have performed it for a number of years, at least several times a week. In special genetic centers, or in hospitals with separate setups for it, that is usually the case. For example, at New York Hospital/Cornell Medical Center, three expert obstetricians perform it day in and day out. The more experienced the doctor, the more reassured you should be. One other advantage of using such a medical facility is the common presence of specialized laboratories, which can more successfully grow the amniotic cell cultures. As an additional reassurance, it's a good idea to ask just what the particular center's complication rate is— to put it plainly, what percentage of the women tested lose their babies within a month of the procedure as an apparent result of the procedure? If the rate is higher than the national average, it might be a good idea to look elsewhere.

You might also ask the center or hospital about the use of ultrasound scanning before amniocentesis, and the availability of qualified personnel to perform the scan. According to current knowledge, the sonogram is a useful procedure (particularly if done *immediately* before the needle insertion, with the patient remaining in the same position). But the unavailability of ultrasound scanning in your area is *not* enough reason not to have the amniocentesis done at all. Such scanning is not essential to a successful amniocentesis.

If you start asking the appropriate questions and making any necessary telephone calls early enough in your pregnancy, you'll have the time to assess the available facilities and to make an intelligent choice. Just as the decision of having amniocentesis done or not should be an informed one, so should the decision of where to have it done.

The Question of Sex

Another decision that faces you and your husband involves the sex of the baby. Can amniocentesis tell parents whether to decorate in pink or in blue, or whether to give away their older daughter's tutus, or whether to prepare their six sons for yet another brother? The answer to the question of sex detection is yes, the baby's sex can be learned through amniocentesis. In fact, that was one of the first things known about the procedure. It was discovered some thirty years ago by Dr. Fritz Fuchs, currently a professor of obstetrics and gynecology at the Cornell University Medical College, and Povl Riis, as they worked together at the University of Copenhagen. When the nuclei of amniotic cells were stained, those from female babies had an additional structure: a Barr body, seen as a dark mass. That structure was not visible if the baby was a male. Nowadays, that information is routinely uncovered in the laboratory analyzing the amniotic fluid, and routinely conveyed to the woman's obstetrician. But obstetricians will not convey it to the parents unless requested to do so. And most obstetricians will not abort a healthy infant simply because it's of the "wrong" sex.

Is it better to know, or to be left in "blissful" ignorance? That depends on a lot of individual factors. One is the depth of a couple's desire to have a child of one sex rather than the other. If it *really* matters to them, whether for deeply rooted psychological reasons, or to break up a string of girls or a field of boys, it may be best to find out the facts during the pregnancy. The couple then has time to adjust to the truth, to come to terms with their feelings, and to accept the sex of their baby before it is born.

Some couples choose to know for practical reasons. They may wish to set up the nursery closets in advance, for example. As one woman put it, "If someone else knows, then we have to know. We both like to be in control of our lives. And since we both work full-time, we figured that it would be easier to get ready if we knew the sex." Sometimes the reason is more fanciful than practical. One pregnant woman couldn't decide, just could *not* decide, whether to ask for the information. Her husband definitely wanted to be surprised at the birth. So her knowing would mean keeping it from him, and keeping it from friends and relatives so that no one would let it slip in front of him. So maybe it would be easier not to know. . . . But then something a friend said turned it for her: "Janey pointed out to me that this would be the best gossip I could ever have. I couldn't resist that." So, in the end, only the new father was surprised at the time of delivery. His wife had managed to keep the news to herself, though she savored the fact that she knew the baby's sex before birth.

Other couples are intent on finding out the news at the same time. One woman, for example, told Kathryn's secretary that she didn't want to get word of the baby's sex over the phone. Instead, she wanted it written down on a piece of paper and placed in a sealed envelope. That night she took the envelope along with her to dinner, and she and her husband opened it together and read it by candlelight. In that way they shared the news in a spirit of excitement and romance.

But many couples opt for complete surprise for them both. Knowing the sex in advance, they believe, would detract from the excitement of the birth, candlelight or no. It may seem not only more exciting to wait, but more natural as well. To some parents, it seems strange to know the baby's sex before the baby's birth, perhaps even a temptation of fate. As one woman explained, "If God wanted you to know, it would be written across your stomach."

Most couples who choose *not* to know the sex beforehand have no regrets about it. But some who know in midpregnancy wish they didn't. It seems, for such parents, as if some of the spontaneity of the pregnancy and birth is gone, that it's all too organized, too businesslike, too "neat." But some couples who "know" may be in for the biggest surprise of all. In rare instances, it is cells from the mother that are mistakenly cultured and examined, instead of fetal cells. It doesn't occur often, because maternal cells have a different appearance than do the baby's cells, but it has been known to happen. And so some couples who are resigned, or delighted, to be having a girl, receive the shock of their lives at the announcement, "It's a boy!"

Unfounded Fears

Once the decision is made to have the amniocentesis done, and to know the sex or not, the waiting begins. As we mentioned earlier, amniocentesis is usually not performed until sixteen weeks after the first day of the last menstrual period, so there is a lot of time to dwell on the procedure. And many mothers do dwell. They worry about the risks entailed for the fetus. They worry about what the test may reveal about the baby they are carrying. They worry about the pain they may associate with the procedure, and the image of the needle that will pierce them. Some couples find themselves worrying alone; they haven't told their families for fear of disapproval, and they don't know what they will tell them if the results are bad.

Once the procedure is over, most couples realize that their worries were needless. They are amazed at how smoothly it went, how relatively painless it was, how efficiently and matter-of-factly it was performed. They often tell Kathryn that it wasn't as big a deal as they expected. There is little advance preparation required, except perhaps to drink a specified amount of water. (A full bladder is important to the ultrasound procedure because it provides a kind of "window" to bounce the sound waves off.) At the genetic or medical center, usually the first thing done after the filling out of forms and changing of clothes is the sonogram. The mother lies down on the table, and oil or jelly is placed on her abdomen. Then an instrument called a transducer is moved over her abdominal area, and the ultrasonic image is projected onto a screen. Usually, the woman is able to see the image. As we described earlier, that in itself is an awesome experience for many mothers-to-be, the first sight of the life they're carrying.

In occasional instances, the woman is then told to get dressed, go home, and come back in two weeks. That's because the sonogram indicated that there is not enough amniotic fluid, or that the pregnancy is not as far advanced as originally calculated. And so the procedure is put on hold. But most often, the sonogram indicates "all systems go," and the amniocentesis proceeds.

Ideally, the woman remains as motionless as possible on the table while the sonogram is being examined and the obstetrician prepares for the "tap" (another word for the insertion of the needle). Some women are a bit unnerved when they see the needle; it is longer than they had imagined. Others are somewhat comforted; they concentrate on how very thin it is. Before the needle is inserted, a sterile solution is wiped on the woman's abdomen to reduce the chance of infection. In some centers, a local anesthetic may also be rubbed or sprayed on, or given by injection (with a very *short* needle). The moment of insertion of the needle for the amniocentesis is rarely as bad as many women have imagined. Most say it's not much worse than a routine injection. As one woman described it, "It was uncomfortable but not very painful.

I've had much worse pain. It's just like a bad shot." The needle is usually left in for less than a minute while the amniotic fluid is being drawn out. It's a time when most women keep their eyes shut, or on the sonogram, or on their husband's face—anywhere but on the place of insertion. In most cases, the needle is then taken out and that's basically the end of it. But a second needle insertion may be necessary if not enough fluid was obtained. (Only rarely are more than two taps done.) In some centers, a second ultrasound scan is then performed to make sure that nothing is amiss, and that the amniocentesis caused no apparent damage.

A small percentage of women require one additional procedure—the injection of Rh-immune globulin. These are the women who are Rh-negative, with Rh-positive mates. Normally during the pregnancy fetal blood doesn't mix with maternal blood, and Rh-immune globulin is administered after the baby's birth to protect any future babies from a dangerous Rh reaction. But during amniocentesis, an accidental piercing of the placenta may enable some of the baby's red blood cells to enter the mother's circulation. The mother may then develop antibodies that would attack the fetal blood cells and endanger the baby. The injection of Rh-immune globulin right after the amniocentesis will prevent such a dangerous immune response.

After the amniocentesis, many women wonder what they were so worried about. Most remember the positives more than the negatives—the fact that it didn't really hurt so much after all, the fact that it gave them an insider's look at their baby-to-be. In many cases, fathers are allowed—and choose—to be present for the amniocentesis, and are most often a reassuring presence. How they react during this procedure can be a clue to how they'll react when the really big day comes. A supportive attitude can give a woman comfort as she contemplates the time when she'll need him even more. "I was quite relieved," one woman recalls, two months after her amniocentesis, some three months before the expected birth. "My husband watched, and at the end he was still standing. So I think he'll make it through the delivery. He didn't even grimace. But he did say something I'll probably hear again: 'I'm glad you're doing this, not me.'" Another woman fears she'll be going through childbirth alone. "Shortly before the amniocentesis, my husband went out to call his office. I didn't see him again until it was all over. He said that he couldn't find the room. I wonder if he'll be any better at finding the delivery room."

In some centers women are advised, after the procedure, to take it easy for the rest of the day and to try to stay off their feet. Normally, there are absolutely no after-effects from the procedure, except perhaps for a black-and-blue mark where the needle went in. Some women do experience a little crampiness, which is definitely nothing to worry about. But about one in eight women experiences symptoms that should be brought to the attention of her doctor, such as a leakage of amniotic fluid, vaginal bleeding, or severe cramps. Such conditions are often just temporary, and may subside by themselves, but they may signal a problem, and your obstetrician should know about them. Also, if you develop a fever—a possible sign of infection—your doctor should be informed right away.

Waiting for Word

While the actual day of the amniocentesis is not a big trial to most women, the weeks that follow are. They are the weeks when she is waiting for the test's results, and feels most in limbo about the pregnancy. Will she be able to continue the pregnancy, confident that the baby is free of Down's syndrome and other less common birth disorders? Or will she find out that she is carrying a seriously damaged fetus? One factor that makes the wait for results difficult is its length—as mentioned earlier, it takes about three to five weeks for the cell culture to be completed and the results analyzed. We're so used to getting test results within a matter of hours, or days, that the wait may seem interminable, especially considering the significance of the results. And if it gets to be past five weeks— which is rare but not unheard of—the couple may worry that that in itself is a signal of a problem. But it just means that the cells are slow in growing, often because of laboratory conditions, *not* that the baby is slow in growing, or that there is any other difficulty with the pregnancy. (As mentioned earlier, if the cells are growing very poorly or not at all, the amniocentesis will have to be repeated to obtain true results. That fact of unsatisfactory growth will generally be known within about two weeks of the procedure.)

During the waiting period, some women try to cope by just going from day to day, and trying not to think about it. But that's not so easy to do. "I tried to forget about it," said one woman, "because when I dealt with it I felt anxious. I kept thinking, 'It will be all right. It will be all right.' But then I thought, 'Will it *really* be all right?' I put it out of my mind, but it was really there. I know it was there because I knew the exact day the doctor was supposed to call." Other women don't even *attempt* not to think about it. In fact, they get deeper and deeper into it, dwelling on the possibilities, and even on the impossibilities. "I got more and more nervous as the time went by," one woman recalled, looking back from the security of good results, and a healthy baby. "I'm so neurotic, I was sure that they would find something else really terrible beside Down's. And I wondered how I would go about having this abortion if I had to. I thought of the pain of it. I'm not a very good patient. And I wondered how I would tell my son. It was a very nerve-wracking time for me. The wait seemed forever. Although I had asked to be told the sex of the baby, that was by far the least important thing."

The wait *is* a long one, and it's better to concentrate on the very strong odds that it will end with the best of news. Many couples call up the genetic counselor during this period to go over their chances and their alternatives. Better to be reminded of the facts, and comforted by them, than to suffer through this substantial period of the pregnancy, a period that should be part of the joy of impending parenthood.

Glad Tidings, Sad Tidings

When the news finally does come, and is the most usual kind— totally reassuring—it is greeted with emotions ranging from restrained joy to uninhibited ecstasy. And with the happiness comes a flood of relief. The baby is free of the chromosomal abnormalities associated with an over-35 pregnancy, and other crippling conditions as well. The couple is free to enjoy the rest of the pregnancy with just the normal worries, like whom to name the baby after. Such relieved parents-to-be are glad that the amniocentesis was done, and willing to have a repeat performance of it should they decide to have a repeat pregnancy.

But what if the news is not good? It can be an emotional blow to any parent, the fact that such a thing could happen in their family, to their child, to them. Why is *this* mother the one of 179, or 105, or 63? It just doesn't seem possible. It doesn't seem fair. But it comes down to the reality that for this couple and this baby, the odds are down to one out of one, and a decision must be made.

For most couples who choose to have amniocentesis, the outlines of this decision are already in place, although the actuality has not truly been contemplated. No one can be fully prepared for the flood of emotions that will sweep over them as they learn of their baby's condition, feelings of rage, of remorse, of self-doubt. How could *I* have produced such an imperfect child? There is also grief, grief for the baby she thought she was carrying, but isn't, grief for the baby who is the true product of the pregnancy. There are other couples, couples who had the amniocentesis not with the possibility of terminating the pregnancy in mind, but simply to prepare themselves in advance for any deformity or disorder uncovered. In that way, they feel, they will have the time, psychologically, to accept the baby's condition, as well as to make any practical arrangements necessary. Some of those couples, however, when confronted with the unhappy reality of the situation, and the impact it will have on their lives, and on this child's life, and on any other children they may have, decide in the end to terminate the pregnancy.

Expectant parents who are the recipients of bad news are generally offered intensive genetic counseling at this point to help them reach a decision they can live with. The abnormality is described to them in detail, along with its likely effect on the quality and length of the child's life. Perhaps most importantly, the parents are reassured that the abnormality is not their fault; the counselor tries to allay the guilt that so many of them feel. "They often want to know if it's something they did that caused it, or whether they could have done anything differently to change the outcome," says Phyllis Klass, the director of the genetic counseling program at New York Hospital/Cornell Medical Center. "We tell them that it's no one's fault. The problem occurred at or prior to the conception, not during the pregnancy. There's no way they could have prevented it."

Because the results of the amniocentesis aren't usually reported until about five months into the pregnancy, the decision about termination cannot be a leisurely one; it generally is made within a few days or a week of the report, if it wasn't made definitively before. The sooner the abortion is performed, the lower the risks involved. Most couples have little idea, before these counseling sessions, just what a midtrimester abortion entails. They didn't want to hear about it unless, and until, they had to face it. In the words of Phyllis Klass, it's "no picnic." It bears little similarity to the dilation and curettage procedure of the first trimester, a procedure some of the women have undergone in previous pregnancies. A D and C is no longer possible because the baby's head is too large; the cervix cannot be dilated enough to remove the contents of the uterus without instruments. Instead, at this more advanced point of the pregnancy, a form of labor is induced by first removing a portion of the amniotic fluid, and then injecting either a highly concentrated salt solution, or prostaglandins, into the uterus. (Prostaglandins are substances produced in all cells of the body, and have a variety of functions. Those that are released naturally by the cells of the uterus cause menstrual cramps and labor contractions.) From the time of the injection, it generally takes about twelve to fourteen hours for the termination to be completed. The termination involves contractions of the uterus, dilation of the cervix, and the expulsion of the fetus and the placenta through the cervix and the vagina. The process is faster if the woman has given birth previously. If it isn't going along well, additional medication may be given, such as intravenous Pitocin, or a prostaglandin vaginal suppository. After the abortion, the woman can generally leave the hospital within a day.

An abortion at this late stage of pregnancy can be a physically and emotionally harrowing experience. It is difficult to go through a process so similar to labor without a healthy baby waiting at labor's end. Yet there are differences from labor. The contractions are not really like labor contractions. The uterus is actually contracting more rapidly, so the pressure is stronger. It's perceived more as a constant state of pain, or pressure, or cramps, than as labor-type contractions that last for a minute and then give some respite. So Lamaze breathing techniques are really not helpful. But pain medication is, and women feel free, in these circumstances, to ask their doctor for pain medication to ease them through the abortion.

Some women like to have their husbands at their side during the abortion for emotional support in this difficult time. They find the presence of their mate soothing and reassuring, and helpful in taking the edge of tragedy off the event. But the husband does not assume the same functions as during a normal labor, when he can coach his wife in breathing and relaxing. There are women who would rather go through this unhappy experience of abortion alone, and save their husband's presence for the joyous occurrence of a healthy birth.

A Time for Healing

There is often a large measure of psychological relief when the abortion is all over. The couple can finally put this difficult experience behind them, pick up the pieces of their lives, and perhaps go on to try again to have a normal, healthy baby. But diving right back into "life as usual," and another pregnancy, might not be such a good idea. There is first a mourning period to go through, the mourning of a vision that has died, and of a baby who never lived. The process of mourning, and healing, can take many months or even a year or more, and that process is best completed before a new pregnancy is started (that is, if the chronological clock so permits). The temptation is strong *not* to wait that long. "Many parents feel that what happened was bad luck, or that they can't do anything right. So they need a new pregnancy to right the wrong, or to prove themselves," says Phyllis Klass, the New York Hospital genetic counselor. "Even if they've already had normal children, they have to prove that they can still produce a normal child. It's a way of wiping the record clean, or restoring their injured self-esteem." But she encourages parents not to give in to the temptation. "Before another pregnancy, it's important to regain emotional and physical health, and to complete the mourning for the lost baby. It's not good for the next baby to be a replacement child, used to wipe out the pain and loss of the other. That child would be expected to make up for the loss and to be special, a very heavy burden. It's best to wait for at least six months, and probably closer to a year, before attempting another pregnancy."

Even if that time period has been allowed, parents are generally very anxious during a subsequent pregnancy, anxious lest they have yet another abnormal baby. They are relieved only when amniocentesis is performed that shows no recurrence of the difficulty. The odds are heavily in their favor for having such good results, and having a perfectly healthy baby. If all goes well, they can finally let go of their heartache and enjoy, at last, the wondrous experience of childbirth and parenthood.

Amniocentesis is the technique that has given these expectant couples and others more options, more control, more knowledge of their growing baby. Over the years, its accuracy and safety have been improved, and work is still being done to make it as perfect a procedure as possible for detecting fetal defects. In one exciting development, a diagnostic technique called chorionic villus biopsy is being tried during the first trimester of pregnancy; it involves taking out through the vagina some cells that would have formed part of the placenta, and analyzing them for clues to fetal maldevelopment. It is performed at eight to ten weeks of pregnancy with ultrasound guidance. This procedure is still strictly experimental, but if it eventually proves out, it will enable earlier, and easier, termination of pregnancy in those cases where it is deemed necessary. For the present, amniocentesis is an impressive, invaluable medical advance, an advance particularly pertinent to women 35 and older. It is an important weapon in diminishing the toll taken, on individuals, on families, and on the society as a whole, by the tragedy of birth disorders.

If you would like to find out about the facilities for amniocentesis available in your community, or within reasonable traveling distance, and you cannot arrange a referral through your physician, you might try contacting one of these national organizations:

March of Dimes Birth Defects Foundation: This organization makes referrals from its International Directory of Genetic Service, which contains listings of centers throughout the world. You might be able to obtain a copy from your local March of Dimes. If not, send a stamped, self-addressed envelope to: Science Information Division, March of Dimes Birth Defects Foundation, 1275 Mamaroneck Avenue, White Plains, N.Y. 10605. Request listings for those centers that are convenient to your area.

The National Genetics Foundation: This organization makes referrals to medical centers throughout the country. It also supplies pamphlets on amniocentesis and genetic disease, and a "Family Health History" questionnaire for a couple to fill out. To obtain information from the foundation, write to: The National Genetics Foundation, Inc., 555 West 57th Street, New York, N.Y. 10019.

8

Your Pregnancy and Your Emotions: The Fears, the Fantasies, and the Facts

The physical changes of pregnancy are dramatic but no more so than the emotional ones. The emotional life of a pregnant woman has been compared to a volcano: All that's been hidden beneath the surface, lying dormant under the tranquility and the everyday concerns of our adult lives, bursts forth in an eruption of feelings and fears, moments of intense ecstasy and times of high anxiety. This emotional eruption certainly can be unsettling, but it is a great opportunity for emotional growth and for taking that important step from woman to mother. The psychological aspects of pregnancy are as meaningful for women over 35 as for younger women, though there are some differences in emphasis. First, this chapter will look at the emotional issues common to most pregnancies, then at the particular concerns of older mothers.

The Good Times

We expect pregnancy to be a time of good feelings, and most pregnant women do experience a lot of them. It's a time that's certainly punctuated by joyful moments, and for some women, a deep sense of well-being pervades the nine months. "I've never been happier" is the way many women remember their period of pregnancy. One expectant mother compared it to being in a state of grace: "It's the best time in my life. Everybody pampers me.

All the attention is on me, and I have a whole new life to look forward to." Another pregnant woman expresses a similar sentiment in different words: "My body is functioning in a way I feel is good, and it supports a life within it." There is commonly a sense of wonder about bringing a new life into the world, a sense of expectancy about what her own life will be like. Some women see their pregnancy as a confirmation of their femininity and proof of their fertility—it is an undeniable sign that they are all woman, and capable of this most womanly of functions.

There is a lot of inward focus at this time, an introspective attitude as women shift their concerns from the outside world to themselves and their pregnancy. It's as if they are consolidating their psychological resources to prepare for the dramatic changes awaiting them. It is a time of replenishment, both physical and emotional. To other people, expectant mothers often seem dreamy and remote, and to their husbands they may seem aloof. But there's a lot going on inside them. During this time you are learning new things about yourself, things you may never have realized, or could never face, before. Any self-knowledge you gain now, either negative or positive, will serve you well as you get ready to take on your most challenging and most rewarding role.

As the pregnancy progresses, involvement with self generally shifts to involvement with the growing baby. What was once but an abstract thought has been transformed into a developing life, a life that is physically entwined with one's own. As you hear the beat of the fetal heart and first feel the movements of the baby within you, the bond between you and your child begins to form.

For Brenda, a woman who was 37 during her first pregnancy, the experience of "quickening" made her feel much more positively toward her baby and much more comfortable with her own condition. "In the beginning of the pregnancy, I felt I had lost control. My thought was that something was growing inside me that was feeding off me, something uncontrollable, something I couldn't stop. But that feeling ended after I felt the baby move. Then I could relate to it as a person. I felt a really close communication with the child. I would talk a lot to her, saying how nice it was in there, how she will become part of our family. I talked to her so that she could get to know me, and so that I could build up a relationship with her."

The positive feelings of pregnancy are important ones, as they help women to put their bodily discomforts and changes into perspective; the emotional highs make the physical lows seem somewhat less devastating and less difficult to cope with. Also, the positive feelings set up a positive attitude toward the baby. They create an environment in which you are receptive to your new child, ready to fall in love with it and to help it grow.

Mixed Emotions

Feelings of euphoria are healthy, and expected, but they are not the whole story. Pregnant women can feel as low as they do high, and don't always understand why. Because of the expectation of constant happiness, they may feel during their low periods that there is something wrong with them, that they are not normal, that their mixed emotions make them somehow unfit to be mothers. In Kathryn's practice, she noticed that many of her pregnant patients were not quite as happy as she would have expected, but she really didn't understand it. She wasn't tuned in to the emotional side of their pregnancies. But Joan Handler, a patient of hers and a clinical psychologist, made Kathryn much more aware of the psychological aspects of pregnancy and better able to empathize with her patients. During Joan's pregnancy, she shared with Kathryn her feelings and emotional changes that this pregnancy had stimulated. She verbalized much of what Kathryn had felt during her own pregnancy but hadn't been able to put into words. Kathryn began to better understand why her obstetric patients aren't always happy. "Women think that pregnancy is supposed to be absolutely marvelous," Joan pointed out. "They are supposed to feel beautiful and think beautiful and anticipate caring for this child with excitement. Actually, women tend to be more isolated and prone to depression during pregnancy. That's not because they're maladjusted or neurotic. Their feelings are perfectly normal, they just don't know it. So patients come in here and say 'No one told me,' or 'I thought that something was wrong with me because of my feelings.' " They may decide that they're unprepared for mothering because of their emotional state. But their emotions are actually very appropriate.

One reason for the misgivings, says Dr. Handler, who had her own son when she was 38, is that pregnancy is such a unique experience. There is absolutely nothing in a woman's prior life that she can relate it to. It is an experience that cannot be undone. Dr. Linda Kestenbaum, a clinical psychologist who works with Dr. Handler, notes that "Pregnancy is the single most irreversible decision one makes in life, more so than the choice of a profession or a mate. Once you make the decision, the child is yours. No matter what, you're always a mother."

With this uniqueness, and this permanence, no wonder most pregnant women feel some ambivalence. Do you really want this baby, after all? Is this the biggest triumph of your life—or the biggest mistake? On a psychological level, there are the conflicting desires during pregnancy to have the baby, and to be rid of it. Since the latter desire is considered unacceptable, it is often translated into dreams, dreams in which anger and resentment are expressed toward the baby. Pregnant women may also dream about being trapped, a reflection of their fears of a more limited lifestyle and of a world made smaller and more restricted by their baby's demands.

Their ambivalence can be troubling to expectant mothers, but it can mean less trouble after the baby is born. Dr. Handler sees ambivalence as a positive force, and its absence as a problem. "I've seen and known women who are totally enamored with the idea of pregnancy and the baby. They haven't dealt with the reality of the changes, and the parts of themselves not ready to assume the responsibility of motherhood. Those women are more prone to difficulty in connecting to their babies." Dr. Handler recalls her own pregnancy as sometimes quite stormy. "My ambivalence was so full blown during pregnancy that when I saw the baby I just fell in love with him. I didn't believe it could feel that good."

Anxiety is another common emotional experience of pregnancy. There is often anxiety over the marital relationships: Will my husband continue to love me, big body and all, or will he pursue a more slender, less pregnant woman? Will I continue to love my husband once I have my baby to love? Financial anxiety is also frequently present during pregnancy. Just as additional expenses come along, with even more being anticipated, one career may be slowing down to a temporary or total halt. More money going out, less coming in, with a whole new person to support, can be a frightening prospect. The whole future can seem frightening, a future filled with new demands and new experiences, a future that will likely be dramatically different from the present. Many women question their ability to cope with such a future, and wonder if they even want to. What will it be like to wake up in the middle of the night to feed a hungry child? What will it be like to have to think twice before going out to dinner or a movie, and perhaps not go at all? What will it be like to combine working outside of the home with mothering, or to give up the outside work for a time? And what will it be like to have the future of a child in one's hands?

More immediate anxiety centers on the well-being of the baby during the pregnancy and its normal, healthy development. There are commonly fears of miscarriage, of birth defects, of something happening that will make the baby less than perfect. Such fears may also be expressed in dreams during pregnancy. Five years after Stacy had her baby, she still remembers waking up in terror. "I started having the dream during the sixth month of my pregnancy," recalls the suburban Philadelphia homemaker. "It began with the birth of a baby girl who looked just like I did in an old photograph. She looked as if she were two or three, the same age I was in the picture. When I looked at her face I was relieved. She looked fine, healthy and pink-cheeked. Then I started scanning the rest of her body. Everything was perfect until I got to her feet. They were crippled and twisted up. I always woke up at that point in a terrible panic. Once my pregnancy was over, and I had a healthy baby boy, I never had that dream again."

The fear of having a less-than-perfect baby is often translated into the attempt to be "perfect" oneself, to avoid harmful drugs, to eat the right foods, to do the right exercises, even to think the right thoughts. Anxiety may be uncomfortable, but it can serve a positive function. It is a signal of the psychological conflicts that are common to pregnant women. Once you are conscious of those conflicts, you can put them into better perspective and face the future with more confidence.

As we can see, pregnancy is not a time when every person feels the same thing, or even when the same person maintains a steady emotional state. It is a transitional time in a woman's life, and her rapidly shifting emotions reflect the impending changes. Pregnant women are noted for the changeability of their moods, a reputation well earned. There are so many things happening to you now, physically, hormonally, psychologically, that each day is likely to bring with it a new way of looking at things. Some women are disturbed by the changeability and the intensity of their emotions. They feel that they are no longer in control of themselves. But others are glad for their newfound ability to express their feelings. One expectant mother recalls how she was trained as a child, and trained well, not to cry. As an adult she had wanted to experience this release, but found it impossible. Her pregnancy has changed that. "I knew I'd feel better about things if I could only cry. Now I'm able to, and it's fantastic. Just this afternoon I felt teary, and I wept, and it felt so good. Finally, I'm unlearning the lessons of my youth."

The changeability may be more difficult for the mate than for the mother-to-be to deal with. He doesn't know what kind of woman will awake alongside him in the morning, or whether she'll react to him with a smile or a sob. But some men see the changes as exciting, and welcome a little unpredictability in their marital lives.

My Mother, Myself, My Baby

During pregnancy, lessons and experiences from your childhood come back in different forms. Conflicts that were created then, and are not yet resolved, may frequently rise to consciousness and force you to deal with them. Conflicts involving one's own mother are the most likely to resurface at this time. Doctors Handler and Kestenbaum explain why: "When you become pregnant, you perceive that you will no longer be taken care of, that this is the end of being mothered for you. Because you anticipate that you'll be on your own, a lot of resentment will erupt, resentment directed to your mother. You start thinking about what you didn't get as a child, what your mother did or didn't do. Another side to this is a competitive feeling with your own mother. You think that you can do better with your child than your mother did with you. That's why most new mothers don't want any interference—that triggers so many feelings. It takes a while before they're secure enough in their own way of being a mother, and don't feel their mother as a threat."

Although things can get worse, for a time, between mother and daughter, ultimately they may get better than ever. For one thing, women come to realize that they can still be nurtured—nurtured by their own children. Psychologists and parents are learning that the mother-child relationship is a two-way street, that the child is not just a taker, but gives back love and care to the mother. A woman who is being nurtured by her child, in a way "mothered" by her child, won't be so angry at her own mother. Dr. Handler tells what happened after she had a child. "At first, I concentrated on the fact that I hadn't gotten what I wanted from my mother. But then I was able to reconnect with her in a special way as I watched her being grandmother to my son. By her giving to my son, it's almost as if she is giving to me." Dr. Kestenbaum emphasizes how pregnancy and parenthood can bring mother and daughter closer. "Although there is anxiety, ultimately a woman will reconnect with her mother through similar experiences. She'll realize, despite the mistakes her mother made, what an incredible role she played in her life." Pregnancy may stretch the mother-daughter bond to its limits, but the parenthood that follows may cement the bond between one mother and, now, another.

A Question of Identity

The emotional states described in this chapter are common features of pregnancy, no matter the age of the pregnant woman. But for the expectant mother 35 or older, there is a somewhat different emphasis, and new elements to consider. Her anxieties, for example, may focus around different issues. She is probably in a more secure financial position, less likely to be thrown by the cost of a larger apartment or the foregoing of a few months' salary. But if she has been collecting that salary for a long time, and has worked hard to establish herself as a career woman, she may be experiencing a different form of anxiety—one focused around that supposedly adolescent but really timeless question: "Who am I?" For most of her adult life she may have been a competent working woman proud of her efficiency, her accomplishments, her reputation among her colleagues as a consummate professional. This professional side of her life has become an integral part of her identity, and perhaps even its very core. And so she may experience her pregnancy as a threat to her sense of self. She may find that she can't work quite as efficiently, or easily, as before, and even when she does, her colleagues may not see it that way. Dr. Barbara Gordon, a psychiatrist, addressed this crisis in identity: "Women often judge themselves on their ability to work in a working world, and pregnancy can be seen as undermining that ability. It's often viewed as an illness, as an inability to function, rather than as a fulfillment. She may also be judged by others by the speed with which she returns to work and by her lack of attention to her children. Such a misguided view sees these women as the only true professional or working women."

Some women solve the identity crisis by not really incorporating first the pregnancy, and then the baby, into their image of themselves or into their lives. But women who do want to get in touch with the experience of pregnancy and motherhood, who want to enhance their lives in this new way, may wonder how well they'll manage it. They *know* they're good at their work, whatever it is they do for a living. They *don't* know they're good at being mothers. And there the anxiety, and the insecurity, lies. "A lot of these women have doubts about themselves as mothers," says Dr. Handler, "and so they go through a whole crisis when they become pregnant later in life. Previously, they've accented the more 'masculine' aspects of their personality. Now they wonder if they can make it as moms, if they have what it takes to function as primary caretakers." But out of this anxiety some women find new joy. After a long time working in a "male" world, being one of the "guys," their pregnancy may represent a reestablishment of their femininity, and an opportunity to put it all together. To them, their pregnancy does not doom them to mediocrity, to impaired performance and to lesser achievements, but rather expands them into new dimensions of themselves, and of life's offerings.

High Expectations

Still, it is hard to give up the standards of the work world, hard not to apply them to the pregnancy. Women who are good at their jobs want to be good at their pregnancies. Women who pride themselves on their rationality in the classroom or the factory or the office want to approach this period of expectancy with equal rationality. But as we've already seen, it can't be so. Pregnancy is an emotional time, a time of dependency, a time of temporarily moving backward into childhood to prepare oneself for one's own child. It can be an especially hard time for women who fight against their feelings. A woman who was 38 when she was pregnant remembers how hard it was for her. "It was difficult for me to accept the anxiety I felt about an experience that every woman who is a mother had gone through. Previously, I had handled conflicts and challenges in my life with a considerable amount of calm. I felt I should be as competent as a pregnant woman as I had been at getting through school. This should be a piece of cake for me. But it wasn't. I wasn't as adultlike as I would have liked. I was childlike and frightened and needy. And I was angry at myself for it."

When things don't run as smoothly, emotionally, as a woman would like, talking to someone in her own situation is helpful. Here is where over-35 women who live in small towns or rural areas may be at a particular disadvantage. They may not know other people who *are* in their situation. (The over-35 first-time pregnancy is largely an urban phenomenon.) Most of the pregnant women they see around the neighborhood may look young enough to be their daughters—and certainly don't seem as if they would understand their concerns. And most of the women who are their age are at a different stage of life, moving toward freedom from family responsibilities, not toward the burdens of caring for a baby. So there may be a strong sense of isolation, of being out of synch with one's generation. Even women who have had babies before may feel it. Rosemary, a woman from a small town in Pennsylvania, had her first baby when she was 30. She made a lot of friends through her child, and never lacked for company for herself or her little boy. But when she had her second baby at age 35, things were different. "The friends I had made before were at a different place than I was. Many of them were thinking of going back to work. They were moving away from home and into the world, while I was going in the opposite direction, giving up my work for a while and my independence. I found I wasn't able to share with them what was going on."

The sense of isolation can be deepened by thoughtless comments, such as "Are you sure, at your age, it's a good idea?" or "You'll be the only gray-haired lady in the PTA." Some of the isolation is self-imposed. Older mothers-to-be may assume that younger pregnant women have no use for them, that they are considered odd and unapproachable because of their "advanced" age. Actually, pregnant women of any age *can* help each other out, can share their joys and their worries with each other, and can provide proof that no pregnant woman is alone in her feelings. When 36-year-old Eleanor met her 20-year-old roommate, she felt more like a parent to her than a friend. As she looked across the room of the community hospital in a small Oklahoma town, she was tempted to dole out motherly advice to the "youngster" in her room. But the "youngster" was a first-time mother, like Eleanor, and soon the two women started talking about their babies, and how to feed them, and about their own aches and pains. By the time they left the hospital they had become friends, despite the age difference, united by their common experience.

The support of others is an important asset in getting over the rough times of a pregnancy. In some communities, health professionals have set up support groups of pregnant women to discuss their experiences and concerns together. Your doctor may know of one in your area. Both private and group counseling can help women deal with the stresses of pregnancy and reach through to the joys. You may decide to set up your own support group with women you've met at an early pregnancy class, or a pregnancy exercise program, or on a tour of your hospital's maternity wing. You can schedule regular meetings over herbal tea to talk over your common concerns and your shared feelings. You'll learn that your feelings are *not* unique, and that you are not alone. No pregnant woman has to be isolated. Although an older woman may be out of synch with most of her peers, she is not out of synch with the rhythms of her own life experiences.

The Perfect Time

For most women who first become pregnant in their late thirties or their forties, this is the very best time for them. Before this time, they just weren't ready. There were too many other things they wanted to do. You may have decided you wanted to see Europe first, or go on an African safari, or at least travel cross-country. You may have wanted the freedom of meeting different kinds of people, and of doing the things you wanted to do *when* you wanted to do them. You may have even devised a kind of mental list of the experiences you wanted to have before becoming a parent. Now that you've done it all (or decided that you *can't* do it all), you can approach childbirth and parenthood with a feeling of greater serenity. Unlike younger women, there's no fear that you've missed something, that your baby is diverting you from more interesting, important pursuits. The search for excitement has given way to the search for contentment, and for the emotional satisfaction that motherhood can bring.

Women today often postpone pregnancy until they get to a certain point in their careers, or achieve a stability in their marriages, or feel more financially secure. The decision to have a child often comes at a time when women are eager for a change—they may have been satiated with a fast lifestyle, tired of a career-centered life, or just tired of their jobs—and want something different, something more human, at the center of their lives. They are ready for a baby, ready to be home more, ready to move out of the fast lane of life, at least for a while. They may be as anxious about the "unknown" as is a younger pregnant woman, but not as resentful when the unknown arrives.

They are at a time of their lives when their values may be changing, and the importance they may have placed on getting ahead has given way to the importance of getting close. Explains Dr. Handler, "They become more interested in affiliation, in closeness, in satisfying their internal needs versus the external gratification of 'making it' in the outside world. They sense that there are other issues to tend to besides just developing themselves careerwise." In deciding to become pregnant, they are consciously choosing to address these other issues and to satisfy these other needs.

That's not to say that as an over-35 pregnant woman you won't feel the ambivalence and anxiety of any expectant mother. But you have the perspective now to understand that this is just a brief stage, and that it will pass into something better. You have also been tested many times before, in many of life's situations, and have likely gained at least some measure of confidence in your ability to make it through to the other side. No, pregnancy is not all wonderful, not a nine-month nirvana of happy feelings and happy thoughts. It is a time when both body and mind are going through enormous transformations, some of them pleasing, some of them distressing. But the biggest transformation is yet to come—the birth of your baby—and it makes all that comes before worthwhile.

9

The Father of the Baby: Your Partner in Pregnancy

You may sometimes feel as if you're in this thing alone. You're in the bathroom throwing up. He's calmly eating breakfast. You're struggling to get your vast bulk out of bed. He's doing his daily bout of push-ups or suiting up for a jog through the park. You feel depressed, agitated, anxious. He seems serene, calm, confident. Why, you may wonder, does he appear so untouched by what's going on around him, so accepting of the changes that are rocking your world? Is it an act, or is it real? What's going on with him, anyway?

What's going on with your mate, during the pregnancy, is likely to be less dramatic than what's going on with you, emotionally as well as physically. And there's a very good reason for it. The pregnancy is not happening to him, nor is the baby changing all his bodily functions to meet its needs. The baby, already so real to you, may remain just an abstraction to him. He may try to deal with it on an intellectual level, reading, asking questions, learning the facts, but have a hard time relating to it emotionally. "The pregnancy really wasn't much," many new fathers claim. "Things went along pretty much as they always do." One man described it as a learning experience for him, not an emotional one. Another compared the nine months to a plateau, a straight line: "There were no spills and no thrills. The whole thing wasn't real until the birth because nothing really happened." It is hard for a man to experience the stages of pregnancy as acutely and dramatically as a woman does. It is hard for him to get in touch with the reality of a life unfelt and unseen. Perhaps that's why the birth itself can hit the father even harder than the mother. The emergence of the infant makes crystal clear what has been going on past nine months as well as what the future holds. It acts as a catalyst for emotions he has not yet fully felt. The man who said he merely "learned" during the pregnancy was much more affected by the birth: "It was a very moving and profound experience. It hit me hard and fast in a joyous way. I was just flooded with tears, and cried for three days. My wife was much cooler than I was."

Does this mean that your nine months of confusion and change-ability will be met by nine months of his coolness, and that only at the birth will he act like the father of your child? While he probably won't be as confused or as changeable as you are during the pregnancy, nor experience quite the same emotional turmoil, he may not be as cool as he puts on, either. There are certain issues that are likely to come up for him now, certain feelings that are quite common to expectant fathers. One feeling is the elation that is part of the emotional package of *both* expectant parents. As one new father recalls thinking, with joy, "I'm making a friend to come into this world." Sometimes it is a more concrete activity that gladdens the fatherly heart. For Brian, the proud new parent of a 15-week-old son, it was, of all things, a shopping spree: "As soon as we found out about the pregnancy, Robin and I went from store to store and bought her a whole new wardrobe of fashionable maternity clothes. When we got home she tried them all on. They looked so funny on her, like limp rags, that we both cracked up at the sight. I never thought she'd grow into them. But she did, and they even got too tight on her. It was fun to watch her grow. It made me aware that something incredible was going on." Watching his wife grow can also make a man proud. Her size is concrete proof of her pregnancy and of his contribution to making her that way. Some men view it as a sign of their virility, of their manliness, and their egos swell along with their wives' bodies.

While most men do not become as introspective as women do at this time, they may spend part of the time in quiet reflection, wondering how this baby will change their lives. Some men, unsure of just how the new baby will fit in, worry as well as wonder about the future. Anxiety is a common state for both mother- and father-to-be, anxiety over their impending change in lifestyle, anxiety over the new roles they will be assuming, anxiety over their new responsibilities. For expectant fathers, in particular, much of the anxiety may center on their financial responsibilities. "How can I afford this thing?" was one man's first thought at hearing the news of the pregnancy. Suddenly, a financial burden that may have been shared between husband and wife seems to have landed full force on his shoulders alone. Even if his wife plans to continue her career, he may foresee time gaps in it, or shortened hours, or lowered expectations—all spelling reduced income. And if she plans to give up her career altogether, he may feel reluctant to question her decision regardless of the limits of his earning potential. After all, how can he deprive his child of the right to be with its mother? And so, afraid of appearing selfish or spineless, he may take on a burden that is too much for him. Even if finances are not currently a problem, many men look to the future and fret about clothing costs, and college costs, and wonder how they'll be able to afford it all. For both rich men and poor men, pregnancy is a time for reappraisal of one's earning capacity and for consideration of how to increase it. As one father-to-be, who's starting his own business, put it, "The pregnancy changed my career goals. I've decided to go for the gold."

Just as your mate may be anxious about his old role of provider, he is also likely to be anxious about his new role as father. He may wonder just how good he can be in this role, a role he may never have played, a role he's never been taught, a role whose possibilities he can't even begin to imagine. Those doubts may be particularly strong in an "older" father who fears that his age will work against him. Will he be energetic enough to play ball with a young son, to go trail-blazing with an older child, to walk his daughter down the aisle? And will he be patient enough to cope with the inevitable demands and frustrations of child-rearing? But balancing those concerns is often the feeling that he can be more rational about both pregnancy and parenting at his "advanced" age, that he is calmer now than he had been a decade ago, that he can put the problems of being a father-to-be and then a father into better perspective. He doesn't have to grow up with his child, but can start out the relationship as a mature man, with the experience of his years to guide him.

Your Mate and Your Marriage

Your husband's years of experience can also help him cope with another common anxiety of the expectancy period—anxiety about his relationship with you, anxiety that you won't be there for him in quite the way you were. It's not hard to understand what would make a man uneasy about his marriage at this transitional time in both your lives. You may act very differently than he's used to as you go through both physical and psychological transformations. What with your tiredness, and your nausea, and your achiness, life together may not seem like so much fun anymore. You may not be up to doing the things you used to do together, and he may not be up to putting up with your endless excuses. He sees things changing in a way he doesn't like, and wonders if you'll ever again be the woman he once knew. Most men attempt to hide any displeasure they feel, but some men don't. "My husband made me feel just awful about myself," one woman recalled, several months after the birth of their second child. "He complained that I wasn't working as hard as I used to, that I couldn't walk as fast, that I was out of shape. He saw me as fat and dumpy, and just destroyed my body image."

A pregnant woman's moodiness doesn't help matters much, nor does her reflective, introspective attitude. Some husbands take it personally, feeling rejected by their wives, seeing their turning inward as a turning away from them, a turning toward the baby. And they may already fear losing their wife to this unborn child. Here is where the maturity of an "older" father can help him to deal with his wife's changes, to see them for what they are, to remain a figure of support rather than of angry rejection. Cary, a 37-year-old news reporter and the father of a 4-month-old son, looks back on the period of pregnancy as a time of great closeness between him and his wife. He believes that his age had a great deal to do with it: "A lot of things that went on would have bothered me ten or fifteen years ago. Many times Phyllis would be withdrawn into herself, or very tired, or unwilling to do anything at all. Sometimes she'd be a little cranky. Sometimes she'd be a little bitchy. When I was in my early twenties, I would have taken it personally. But at this time in my life I was able to understand what was going on."

But even older fathers, even fathers who don't feel like outsiders in their marriage, may feel like outsiders to the experience that their wives are going through. Certainly, there's a lot of it they don't *want* to know about firsthand—the fatigue, the discomfort, and finally the pain—but they would like to know that they still do count, that their importance did not end with the act of conception.

Sometimes, it is the wife who discounts the male's importance in the pregnancy process. As one man recalls the attitude of his first and former wife, "Her message to me was 'You did your bit, buddy. Now just get out of the way. There's no real role for you here.'" In other instances it is something that the man feels within himself, reinforced by society's attitudes. He doesn't quite know how to participate in the pregnancy experience in a real way; he has been taught that the role of the father-to-be (and then of the father) is a peripheral one, and so he settles into it with just a vague sense that he is missing out on something important.

His feeling of exclusion can be further fueled by someone who has taken on a primary role in his pregnant wife's life: her obstetrician. Most often a man, this doctor is privy not only to his wife's body but to all the emotional changes she's going through. If the husband is in some ways an outsider, the obstetrician is in every way an insider, a vital link in the pregnancy and the birth of the baby. He sees the woman at least once a month. He listens to the baby's heartbeat. They talk together about everything relating to the pregnancy. Many women experience some awe and "in loveness" with their obstetrician, and an important relationship develops between them. The husband may feel left out. He may feel as if he has to compete with the doctor for his own wife.

Just as the husband is jealous of the doctor, his wife may be feeling her own pangs of jealousy—jealousy of every woman who still has a waistline and normal-sized breasts, of every woman who she thinks may catch her husband's eye. The word has gotten around that expectant fathers are especially vulnerable to extramarital affairs, and their wives may fear the worst. This flight to another woman, some people have said, is part of a general pattern of flight—flight from the responsibility of impending fatherhood, flight from their wives' neediness, flight to more appealing pursuits (and more attractive women). Actually, any flight that occurs is generally more fanciful than real. Men may *think* of getting away, but in most cases stick it out. As one frightened father-to-be describes it, "I was so psychologically uncomfortable I did feel like getting away. I wanted to escape, to pick myself up and get the hell out. But I knew that I was really a part of it. I resolved that there would be no turning around. This is it. I'll deal with it from here. I'll live with it and work it out." The fantasy of flight is common to both expectant fathers and mothers, but for men it may become more powerful because of their feelings of not really being needed anyway. They may suspect that the only role they will serve in their new family is that of provider—a role they would love to escape from. But their most common real-life response is to try to carve out a more meaningful role for themselves, to move closer to the family, not further away. "If anything, there is an even greater commitment to the wife and to the family during this time," points out Dr. Handler. "The male's struggle is to be part of the new unit." He may dream of faraway places, but his heart remains at home.

As men struggle for ways to be included in the tumultuous but tantalizing experience of the pregnancy, their psychological desires may be translated into physical fact. Approximately one in ten expectant fathers report such familiar-sounding symptoms as nausea, morning sickness, stomach distress, and even abdominal bloating, conditions that often appear about the third month of his wife's pregnancy and subside a short time before or soon after the delivery. They are symptoms that provide tangible evidence of the man's strong identification with his pregnant mate and of his effort to be part of what is going on. The expectant father cannot carry new life within him, but he has helped to create it, and his body is making it clear that he will not be shunted aside.

Like Father, Like Son?

There is another type of identification process that commonly occurs in expectant fathers, and parallels the experience of their wives. As we discussed in chapter 8, pregnancy is a time when many women reexamine their relationships with their own mothers, and begin to identify more closely with them as their roles are about to coincide. Men begin to dwell on their fathers, sometimes in admiration, and with the determination to use the father as a model of good parenting; in other cases in anger, and with the determination to be a very different kind of father. Many "older" expectant fathers tend toward the latter feeling because of the pattern of fathering that was prevalent thirty and forty years back—fathering that was often quite passive, that left most practical child-care to the mother, that sometimes left a legacy of bitterness in the sons. Matthew, a man raised in the 1940s, tells what it was like for him then, and how he hopes it will be different for his child of the 1980s: "My father wasn't exactly mean, but he didn't play an active part in doing things with me," says Matthew, who thought a great deal about his father during his wife's recent pregnancy. "We never played football together, we never went fishing together. He wasn't an active participant in my life. He was never open with me, so I couldn't be open with him. I didn't feel I could say 'Hey Dad, could I talk to you?' or 'Let's go and play some ball.' But I want my son to be able to shoot the bull with me. I want to have a nice easy-going relationship with him. And I want to give him what my father never gave me. I'm not talking about material things. My father was generous with those. I'm talking about the love and affection that I never knew from him."

For some men, the pull of the past is too strong to break away from. They *want* to do things differently, but they can only repeat what they've grown up with. "There is a tendency to recapitulate one's own upbringing," says Dr. Kestenbaum, "which generally means feeling and being on the outside. Most of today's new fathers were raised in traditional families, where mother was the focal point and father a less significant figure. He was almost a recessed figure, either not there at all or experienced as withholding and inaccessible. That has caused pain for a great many men. They often feel that they want to do it differently, to be a more significant parent to their child. Such a man may be terrified that he is going to emerge as a gray figure in the background, like his father, because that's his only association. His terror is that he won't exist. He doesn't want to repeat his father's role of nonexistence, but he has no male role models to combat it."

A New Kind of Father

Despite the difficulty of taking an independent stance, and of shedding their father's influence, more and more men are doing just that, imprinting their own style on their relationship with their children. And they are doing it early on, during the pregnancy, showing that they are *not* cut from the same cloth as their fathers. In fact, a study of 156 expectant fathers revealed that the men who were dissatisfied with their own fathers during childhood were more highly involved with their wives during the childbearing period and closer to their infants after the birth. These men were apparently determined to be the kind of father that they themselves never knew. The growing involvement of fathers has become apparent at every stage of the pregnancy, starting with the first visit to the doctor, when many men go along to meet the physician, to gain an understanding of the medical aspects of the pregnancy, and to ask their own questions of this professional who will be so important in the months ahead. Some men don't miss any of the doctor's appointments, while others reserve their visits for such "highlights" as the amplification of the fetal heartbeat, possible at about the eleventh or twelfth week of the pregnancy. Such participation gives the father the feeling that he is an important part of the pregnancy, that his wife and his doctor don't have a "special thing" going that excludes him, that the baby she is carrying is not hers alone. It can also serve a less lofty function. Says one new father, "Going to the checkups was a way of my being part of the whole experience and of showing my wife moral support. It was also a good excuse to get off from work." (This was a father especially elated toward the end of pregnancy, when he found himself going to the doctor's office more, and to his own office less.)

The mates of women over 35 often have another point of connection with the pregnancy experience and the growing baby—the amniocentesis. Not only is this an opportunity for a man to be emotionally supportive of his wife, but also to witness the reality of the life growing within her. He can see the baby's form on the sonogram, hold his baby's likeness in his hands as he gazes at this most miraculous of all photographs—the sonographic image of his unborn child. When he learns the results of the amniocentesis, the baby may come even more alive to him. "At that point I knew the baby was all right. I knew his name, I knew his sex," says Chuck, who became a proud father four months ago. "Ever since that time, someone's been living here with us in one sense or the other."

There are other channels for involvement, including couples

groups in some communities, in which both expectant mothers and fathers are invited to share some of their feelings about becoming new parents. The assumption is that the men as well as the women are going through changes, and need a forum to explore them. Now available in virtually all communities are "preparation for childbirth" classes, programs that will be discussed in great detail in the next chapter. But they are relevant to this chapter also in that they focus on the couple, with the father's importance much more than a symbolic one. He is given the place he should have as that of an equal partner in the childbirth experience, though with a different role than his wife's. Your husband may find his inclusion frightening at first and may even balk at your attempts to take him along to class, but his fright will almost inevitably turn to fascination as he becomes steeped in the rituals and realities of childbirth.

For men who are "older" fathers, and who have had a previous child a number of years back (perhaps by a previous marriage), the differences from their past experiences are obvious. This is what they looked like to Paul, the 36-year-old father of an 8-year-old and a newborn: "Both my children were born at the same hospital, but the practices of the hospital and the obstetrician and the nursing staff were very different. The role of the father was more liberal this time. It included more involvement. The hospital staff really wanted me to participate in all the decisions, a far cry from eight years ago, when they grudgingly permitted me to know what was going on." As men become more involved in both the pregnancy and the childbirth, they are gradually preparing themselves for the fatherhood that awaits them. It is a time for your mate to acclimatize himself to his new role, to slowly transform himself into the father he wants to be. With this preparation, the shock of the birth will be less traumatic for him, the demands of new parenthood less difficult to meet.

The cultural changes in the role of the father-to-be are clear, but each couple meets them in a different way. The best way is to approach the childbirth experience as an adventure in sharing, as an opportunity to make important decisions together. To be truly equal partners means to have a dialogue about as many of the issues and decisions involving the child as possible—about the choice of obstetrician versus midwife, hospital versus maternity center, even breast-feeding versus bottle-feeding. The baby you are carrying is your mate's baby, too, and his feelings regarding its welfare should be acknowledged. That doesn't mean that his word is the last word, but that his views should be given equal weight with yours. The art of compromise comes in handy here—an art that many over-35 couples are quite practiced at, and that will stand them in good stead.

The "Mother" in the Man

But the focus on equality does not mean that differences should be overlooked, and as we mentioned earlier in this chapter, there are differences in the pregnancy experience for men and for women. The physical ones are obvious, the emotional ones subtler but just as real. Women are more volatile during this time, more dependent, more needy. And what they need is what their mates are in a perfect position to give them. This is a time when men can get in touch with the mothering part of themselves, and nurture the future mother in their lives. "The pregnant woman needs to feel mothered and taken care of," point out Doctors Handler and Kestenbaum. "She feels ambivalent, vulnerable, overwhelmed by her own conflicts about mothering. This is the perfect opportunity for the man, who is calmer at this time, to really move in and be a good mother to his wife. A lot of couples are reluctant to let the woman become that dependent at a time she's supposed to be self-sufficient, or to let the man be the mother he's able to be. But it can be achieved, and is the mark of emotionally successful pregnancies and marriages." Dr. Handler tells how it happened during her own pregnancy. "When I was eight months pregnant I broke my ankle. I remember looking up at my husband from my wheelchair and saying 'Why did I do this?' He shrugged his shoulders, smiled, and said 'I guess you needed to be my baby for a while.' That is what both of us allowed me to become. I felt very little, and dependent, and in need of a mother, which he thoroughly enjoyed being. There is a place for that kind of nurturing in a marital relationship."

It certainly makes the man feel important, a source of strength to both his wife and unborn child, an emotional as well as biological partner in the creation of life. It also helps him to get in touch with that part of himself—his capacity for nurturance—that will be called upon soon not by dependent mate but by dependent child. Once your husband has learned the pleasures of being more than a financial provider he will be eager to experience those pleasures again as a fully participating parent. Most directly, his ability to give to you at the time you need it, and your willingness to take from him, will help to cement your relationship in preparation for this new phase in your lives. After the birth, it may be your husband who needs more of the "mothering," and you who nurture him for a time. As the love and care flow from one of you to the other, as your sensitivities to each other's needs sharpen, your marital relationship can more than survive the birth of a baby. It can flourish, with each of you enhanced by the experience, with a new alliance formed between you to welcome your new baby in unity and with love.

10

Your Pregnancy and Your Profession: Meeting the Challenges, Planning the Future

A woman's first thought when she finds out that she's pregnant is likely to be how she will break the news to her husband. Her second thought may be how she will break the news to her boss. Chances are that she expects a considerably less elated response from her employer than from her husband. Even if her employer's words are appropriately congratulatory, she may fear a condescending undertone, a note of disappointment that all her hard work has come to this, that she will be exchanging her role as a professional for that of a parent. Although pregnant women are becoming more accepted in the work force, and attitudes toward them are becoming more enlightened, unfair or irrational responses to pregnancy among working women are still common enough to keep most pregnant women quiet about their condition until their claims of overeating lose credibility. They fear that they will no longer be taken quite as seriously and that their jobs will be viewed as being up for grabs. And they fear that they might actually lose their position, although it's illegal.[1]

One woman, pregnant for the second time, finally told her boss. His response: "What an abomination!" The next day, at a staff meeting, he introduced his employees to a visitor, listing their functions. The introductions went like this: "Bob does our market research. Carol handles our public relations. And Bonnie makes babies." That incident occurred about five years ago, but similar incidents are not uncommon even today. Another man describes his response to his pregnant employees: "I ask them why they can't decide between a career and a family."

Many of Kathryn's patients tell of a negative response at work to the news that they are pregnant—a response that comes from some female employers as well as from some males. She herself was fortunate enough not to have that experience. She was a third-year resident in obstetrics and gynecology when she became pregnant with her son. It was a very male-oriented program with few female participants, none of them pregnant. Kathryn was concerned about the reaction to her pregnancy, and how she would be treated, so she kept her condition a secret for almost six months. (Those white coats do come in handy.) But it got to the point where she could no longer camouflage her expanding waistline, and even the white coat started to bulge. One weekend there was a tennis match for the residents—calling for sporting attire rather than bulky coats—and Kathryn knew that the time to tell had come. The Monday morning after the party she walked into her department chairman's office and told him, in a straightforward way, that she was pregnant. He said, "Gee, my wife asked me after the party if you were pregnant, and I said 'No, of course not!'" But he was fine after that, and Kathryn was never treated

1. In 1978, Title VII of the Civil Rights Act of 1964 was amended to include the Pregnancy Discrimination Act. Under this act employers are required to treat pregnancy and pregnancy-related medical conditions the same as any other medical disability in administering employment practices and health benefits. If you believe you have been discriminated against in any way on your job because of your pregnancy, you may file a charge of discrimination at any field office of the U.S. Equal Employment Opportunity Commission (EEOC). These offices are located in 49 cities throughout the United States and are listed in local phone directories. You may call an office collect if you believe you have an employment discrimination complaint or charge against your employer.

any differently than she had been before by him or by the other residents.

The best way to deliver the news is in a straightforward way, with a discussion of your future career plans as well as you can predict them. Apologies are unnecessary and unwise, but some women do give them. One employer related, "Sometimes a woman would come in here and give me a long story, how she didn't plan to have a family, but there was a failure of birth control and she's pregnant, and she'll have the baby even though she's miserable about it. I'd much rather a woman just tell me the facts, without the embellishment." It's a good idea, before you inform your boss of the situation, for you to find out your company's policies on such issues as maternity leave, disability benefits, health insurance coverage, and the exact status of your job after time out for a baby. In that way you'll be able to discuss your plans more intelligently, and perhaps even suggest a change in existing procedures helpful to you and your employer.

Even women who are themselves in the position of hiring and firing can experience prejudices toward pregnancy. While conducting a job interview, one woman was struck by something in the applicant's attitude. She sensed that he saw this as his big opportunity—that since she was pregnant, she must be on her way out, and her job would be his for the taking. A woman who has clients or patients may find their attitude equally distressing. Fearing abandonment, the client may be angry or disapproving, and question whether the pregnant woman can handle both her business and her baby.

For a woman over 35 who is well established in her career, those attitudes may be compounded by surprise. You are perceived as a "working woman," dedicated to your profession, past the time when a family would seem a likely contender for your time and attention. Your pregnancy may seem out of character both to your coworkers and your employer. You've gotten this far, why put it all on the line for a baby? But your age and experience also provide you ammunition against those who would lay your career to rest. You have probably established yourself by this time as a valuable member of your company, and care would be taken to accommodate any new needs you may have so as not to risk losing you. From this position of relative power, you have more options open to you and won't be easily forced down the career ladder you have so painstakingly climbed. You probably have the acumen to handle negative comments. You are a person of importance now, a person of maturity, and you are unlikely to allow your pregnancy to detract from your accomplishments.

But you do have to deal with what's going on outside of you—and what's going on inside of you. Just as people may treat you as if you're not quite as competent as you were, not able to get the job done, you may sometimes feel that way about yourself. After a bout of morning sickness or a night of insomnia, you may stagger into the office with anything but work on your mind. Knowing how to deal with such ailments (see chapter 3) will help you to keep them from interfering with the day's work. But you may have to alter your daily schedule, for example, by keeping off your feet toward the end of pregnancy, snacking during the day, or making more frequent trips to the restroom. Finding some time to rest during the day, preferably by taking a short nap during the lunch break, would also keep your spirits and your productivity up. Some women don't like to slow down even a little bit, but you can cut back on shopping or evenings out, rather than letting the quantity or quality of work suffer.

Unless your job is physically stressful or poses hazards to the baby, it is medically acceptable for you to work right up to the due date, or even beyond if the baby is late. (If your pregnancy is a complicated one, you will want to ease off toward the end of your pregnancy, as discussed in previous chapters.) Many women keep right on working, going from one form of labor to another with no time in between. Dr. Joan Handler, the psychotherapist and mother of a young son, remembers her own determination to keep going until the very end. "I assumed that there was no reason I should stop working in advance. I was literally in the middle of a therapy session when I went into labor." Some women who worked until the end regret it afterward. They feel that they missed the time to wind down, to prepare themselves psychologically for the birth, to enjoy this last bit of time they had to themselves. But others prefer to remain active rather than sitting around waiting. Every woman should make the choice for herself. You should evaluate not only your physical and financial condition, but also your emotional needs, before deciding when to pack up your papers and make the move home.

Having a Baby, Ending a Career?

An even more difficult decision involves deciding whether to continue working outside the home after the baby is born. In fact, it may be one of the most important issues you must deal with at this time, and the most difficult to resolve. It's often made no easier by pressures from family, friends, and colleagues. A pregnant woman is often told by a well-meaning relative that her career in the workplace should give way to her career as a mother. To do anything else is not to be a real mother, she's told; it is to put her family in jeopardy and her child at risk. Why have a child at all if you won't be home to take care of it? And so the pressure is on to chuck her career, to rip up her resume, to trade in her traveling case for diaper case and become a full-time mom.

But before she can decide whether to relent or resist, a pregnant woman will often feel a different kind of pressure, pressure that has become more powerful as women have made more professional inroads. It is the pressure of the work world and its inhabitants, pressure telling her that she must keep going without pause, that her baby is an inconvenience to be shunted aside, that she will only be rewarded as long as she produces; if she quits, or even takes a breather, it's an indication that she is not made of "the right stuff," and that her years of work have been in vain. "The working world demands your return," says Dr. Barbara Gordon, New York psychiatrist and mother of two. "Women often succumb to the demands because their major gratification has been from their work. It has been the source of their identity." Dr. Gordon points out that it is not only a woman's male colleagues who pressure her to "stay the course"; her female coworkers may be even more demanding. "Women who don't want to mesh work and child-rearing often look down on those who do. They're the worst offenders in this. They're not home with their children, so they don't want anybody else to be either. It's a form of jealousy."

Some women also experience social pressure to continue working. Their work has provided them with an exciting image and social presence. They have gone beyond the traditional limits of their sex and are sought out for their daring and their worldliness. But if they give it all up for the nursery, who will want them for cocktail banter or for dinner party philosophizing? Who will want to hear about the latest sale on diapers, or the merits of various baby foods? For fear of seeming less exciting, less socially desirable, even downright boring, they may lean toward keeping the job they love to talk about, even if they don't love the job itself.

Three Women, Three Decisions

Different women cope with the competing pressures in different ways, ultimately reaching their own resolution. Here we'll meet three women who went in different directions, making very different decisions during pregnancy about their work lives and their babies.

Gwen, almost 39 and halfway through her first pregnancy, has just been promoted to a very important position in the public relations firm she works for. If she was undecided before, the promotion made up her mind for her—she is first and foremost a career woman, and the baby will fit into her life as a working woman. "The pressure is on me now to perform, and I intend to prove that I can do it. I am going to take a short time off after the birth—about six weeks in order to get back in shape physically—but then I'll be back to work full-time and more. If I decide to nurse, it will only be for about a month. As a career woman there are certain shortcuts you have to take, and one of them is breast-feeding. Sometimes I think it's unfortunate that my husband and I both have such demanding careers, and that we're at crucial points in terms of time demands. The baby may get short shrift for a while, but I hope that it will eventually even out."

Dina's pregnancy caused her to slow down rather than speed up her career. It is a decision that she spent two years mulling over, and only when she resolved it did she go ahead with the pregnancy. "It took me that much time before I could accept and feel good about it," says the 35-year-old bank executive. "But some of my superiors still don't understand. How could a 'fast track' person like me decide to stay at the same level for several years?" Dina has spent much of her career working fourteen- and sixteen-hour days, "putting my life on the line for the bank to get ahead." But she doesn't plan to continue at that pace after the baby is born. "I won't be the one who's always there. I'm not going to work at night. I'm not going to travel. I'll be an eight-hour-a-day person. I decided that I just can't do it all. I can't be A-plus at everything.

I'd rather be A or B as a mother and simply adequate at work."
Dina plans to take her "slowdown" even one step further, working
a four-day week. Her husband also plans to work only four days
so that they each will have more time to spend at home with the
baby. Dina believes that her long experience at the job will allow
her to arrange her hours as she wishes. "That's an advantage of
working here so long. I know more people and have more options.
It would be difficult to look for a new job and get one for four
days." By having waited to have her baby, Dina hopes to have
more time to spend enjoying motherhood, and the joys that only
a baby can bring.

Dr. Handler, the third woman in this section, is a woman we
have met before, one who made an important decision during
pregnancy and can report on how it turned out. Dr. Handler had
been doing adjunct teaching and private psychotherapy when, in
her seventh month of pregnancy, she was offered a full-time teaching job that would begin right after the birth. Her first reaction
was: "Fantastic, I'll take it." Then she had second thoughts and
asked her husband for his opinion. His reaction: "It's totally up
to you, but you've got to be psychotic to do it." She figured out
what her life would be like if she took the teaching job—out of
the house forty or forty-five hours a week, preparing for her classes
much of the time she was home, and squeezing in child care. It
took her a long time to reach a decision because the job was very
appealing to her, but she finally opted against it. "I wanted both.
I wanted the job and time with the baby. I knew I would be
deprived either way. But I came to realize what was most important
to me—spending those first few years with my child. I figured that
if I overwhelmed myself I would miss out on the fun of mothering."
She has no regrets about turning the job down. Now, four years
later, her life as a mother and as a professional are both on track.

Some professionals who work with pregnant women perceive
that it is usually the "older" mother, such as Dr. Handler, who is
more willing to slow a career down in exchange for more time with
the baby. One reason has already been touched on: The woman
over 35 is likely to be more secure in her career, and freer to take
time off without penalty. But there is another factor at work, as
Dr. Linda Kestenbaum, clinical psychologist, explains: "These
women are at a different point in their lifespan. They can see that
they have less time ahead of them, less overall time to spend with

their child. As a result, they tend to want to take fullest advantage of the time they have. They're aware of what's packed into the next twenty years, and they're aware of their own mortality. So their willingness to make career sacrifices is related to their maturity and to their ability to look at their mortality."

There are clearly many options open to career women that should be considered during pregnancy. Some women intend to continue their careers full-time after the birth, returning to the job after only a few weeks or few months at home. Others take a longer period off, a year or more, perhaps even until the child is old enough for nursery school or kindergarten, and then resume a full-time job. That type of break for child-rearing is considered much more acceptable for women than for men (unless the women are in a high-technology field where their skills might quickly become obsolete). Women who have been working more than full-time, such as Dina, the banker, often determine to slow down to a less hectic forty-hour week. Women who have been driving themselves hard at the job are often relieved at letting up on that part of their lives, and enjoying the pleasures of home and family. As we learned, Dina intends to take that one step beyond, reducing her paid work to four days a week. (It's important to note here that women who stay home with their children are also working women; they just don't get paid for what they do).

Other options opening up for working mothers include flexitime (flexible working hours) and job sharing (dividing a job between two employees). As employers are realizing how beneficial such arrangements are, both for the workers and the company, they are being made more available to women who want both career and family. Some employers are even establishing formal job-sharing programs. An ambitious one has recently been instituted by the New York State Department of Law. Originally, such arrangements were limited to clerical and secretarial workers, but job sharing is spreading to middle management and the professions. (New Ways to Work is a community-based organization in San Francisco that provides information about job sharing and other job-related innovations; there may be a similar group in your area.)

Still another alternative—part-time work—is ideal for many women who want the best of both worlds. Women who can find such a position (either by rearranging their current job or by working at another, more amenable, firm), and who can afford the reduction in salary and benefits, are often quite happy with this blend of office and home life. Anne, a patient of Kathryn's, worked many years as a social worker in an adoption agency before she became pregnant. She didn't want to give up her work—or the opportunity to participate fully in her baby's care. She asked the agency to consider carefully what they told their own adoptive mothers: that a baby needs a caring *and* available parent. In other words, practice what you preach. She was apparently quite persuasive. She went on a three-day-a-week schedule, doing paperwork at home the other two days, and being available to watch and help her baby grow.

In thinking about the future, there is another person to consider—the father. Although it is still far from the norm, some fathers are choosing to make their own career sacrifices, either by reducing their working hours or by staying home full-time with their child as the primary caretaker. Such decisions afford more flexibility to the mother, and more peace of mind if she continues to work outside the home. Couples can tailor such arrangements to their own needs and to the demands of their respective professions. Perhaps, in the future, men will not be as heavily penalized in the work world as they generally are now for taking on a primary parenting role, and more couples will be free to choose this option.

Choosing Child Care

Who will take care of the baby while you are at work? Again, there are various possibilities to consider. Some women have a relative who is willing and perhaps even eager to take on the responsibility. If this person is warm and responsive to the child's needs, this can be the ideal arrangement; the child will be tended in its own home by a loving caretaker. Other women hire a child care helper to substitute for them while they're away; if they choose the person with great care, that too can work out well. Sometimes the helper is a neighbor who is staying home with her own children. If she has the time and love for more than her own, your child can benefit from her experience as a mother as well as from the built-in playmates. Other alternatives such as family day care and day care centers exist in most communities. All such arrangements should be checked out very carefully beforehand, and monitored to make sure that they are working out satisfactorily. Before you make any child care decisions, it is a good idea to ask other mothers in your community about the choices they've made, and how they've turned out. Benefiting from other people's experiences can help guide you to what's right for you, and help you to avoid making emotionally costly mistakes.

Before you hire anyone to care for your child, you should interview the candidate, check out references, and observe his/her interaction with the baby. The personal feeling you get from talking to the caretaker may be one of your most important clues to his/her suitability. But you may find that the first person you hire won't be the right person. The first woman Kathryn had care for her son was a grandmotherly 68-year-old who had a lot of experience with babies. She did very well with Kathryn's son until he began to walk. Then, he became too much for her. He was so active she couldn't keep up with him, and she quit before he ran her totally ragged. The warm and loving woman who is wonderful with babies and toddlers may not necessarily be the best one to face the discipline problems of a 6-year-old. Children need stability, but they also need someone appropriate for their particular stage of development. If you're lucky, you'll find someone who can make the transition with your child; otherwise, you may have to change caretakers every few years.

Even after you've hired someone for the job, it's a good idea to try to observe him/her in action once in a while. You might try dropping in unexpectedly upon occasion, or arranging a group activity for the family and the caretaker. This person is important to your child's early development; it's important that he or she guide it as you would like, and that he or she and the baby form a warm and healthy relationship.

Some mothers are afraid that the relationship will be *too* warm— that their child will become more attached to the caretaker than to them, and that they will be left out in the cold. But a babysitter can never truly take a mother's place. Yes, the child will likely come to love the babysitter. Yes, the bond between them may well be an important one that provides the child with a feeling of security. Those are all positive outcomes, proof that the parents have made a wise choice of caretaker. But you are always the mother and your child will not be likely to forget.

Breast-Feeding and Working: You Can Do Them Both

Still another decision that most mothers make during the pregnancy involves breast-feeding. For a career woman, it's an especially important one to make fairly early on because it affects working arrangements after the birth. Most businesses do not allow nursing at the office, so a potential conflict is set up for women who want to breast-feed their babies and still maintain their careers. But the conflict can be resolved.

The general trend, which had been toward bottle-feeding, began to reverse in the 1970s toward breast-feeding as more women came to recognize psychological, nutritional, and immunological benefits. But how do those compare to the psychological and financial benefits of a career? More and more, women are finding that they do not have to sacrifice one for the other. You can nurse your baby and still go to business, though you have to have the determination to make it succeed. It's best if you can stay home to breast-feed for the first three months of the baby's life in order to get the "machinery" well established and the feeding rhythm properly developed between mother and baby. When the baby is six or seven weeks old, it's a good idea to provide a supplementary bottle at least once a week to get the baby accustomed to this form of feeding. Once work outside the home is resumed, pump your breasts at least once during the day, either by hand or mechanical pump. (For more information on hand expression and on pumps, contact La Leche League in your area, a group that gives support and advice to nursing mothers.)

If there's a refrigerator at your office, you can express the milk into a sterile container and save it to be given to the baby the next day. Otherwise, the baby can have formula for the midday meal. Women who nurse on a part-time basis should try to breast-feed the baby for at least the early-morning and late-evening feedings. Those are the major feedings, and it's difficult to pump out all the milk that's been built up for them.

If you plan to stay home for only a month or two after the delivery, you may have particular doubts about breast-feeding. Is it any use, if it's for so short a time? The answer is yes, even a brief period of breast-feeding, which provides the baby with valuable antibody protection, is better than none at all. And many mothers who start out rather warily, planning to give up nursing rather quickly, decide that they want to continue breast-feeding on the part-time basis described above. Breast-feeding provides a working mother and her baby a wonderful opportunity to come together after a long day apart, to shut the rest of the world out and share the warmth and intimacy of this most special relationship.

After the Birth

Just as feeding plans may change once the baby is on the scene, other well-laid plans may also fall by the wayside. Things may just not work out as you intended. That is commonly what happens to women who think they can go on as they did before. They try to keep up their work life, their social life, their recreational life, and find that it all begins to collapse around them. Dr. Kestenbaum of New York recalls, "I worked until the day I gave birth. Then I took just three weeks off, and resumed my practice and my teaching. My son was colicky and was up virtually twenty-four hours a day, so my husband and I took two-hour shifts at night. Basically we got no sleep. At the end of three months I had the feeling 'I hate my life.' " She says that she felt totally overwhelmed because she tried to function at her previous level in every area. "That's impossible to do. You just can't 'do it all' toward the end of pregnancy and for the first three years of a child's life. Women who try to do everything often develop anxiety and end up in therapy. The idea is to accept that in certain areas of your life you'll function at fifty percent instead of ninety-five percent. You can feel good about yourself without having to prove yourself in every aspect of life."

A patient of Kathryn's who has two children was also surprised at what happened after her first baby was born. Her intention while pregnant was to have the child, go back to her work as a psychiatrist, and hire someone to take care of the infant. She thought there would be absolutely no interruption of her work. But she found that that plan was "crazy," at least crazy for her. "I had really been gung ho about my career, but after my daughter's birth my ambition went to pot. My career just took second place. I still worked long hours outside the house, but never full-time since then, and I cut out my private practice." Does she regret it, now that she's nine years down the road? "I regret that I didn't spend even more time with my children. I didn't have the stamina or the courage to say 'Screw the world, I want to be with my kids.' I was too afraid that my career would be damaged. Now I regret some of the housekeepers I had. I should have been there instead. Children grow up and then you can work, for years and years and years. But they are only young once. Yes, it's possible to find an adequate replacement while you're working, but as a mother you should recognize how much you can give to your children, and just how important you are to them."

Women who do resume a full-time career shortly after the birth soon realize the difficulties that can be involved—trying to put in a full day's work after almost a full night up with the baby, a babysitter who leaves you in the lurch, a sick child whom you don't want to leave. Another potential problem—the problem of guilt at leaving the baby in someone else's care—is often initially resolved by the thought that it's the quality of time spent with the child, not the quantity, that's important. But then many women come to realize that the quality is not always so wonderful after a high-pressure day at work, especially if things didn't go well that day. It's not so easy to leave office problems at the office. Some women respond to the pressure by quitting their jobs and staying home full-time with their baby, even if this wasn't their original plan. Cara had worked for ten years as a technical illustrator for a Detroit automotive firm when she became pregnant for the first time. She had always considered herself a career person, and didn't see that changing with motherhood. But she soon found that combining her old career with her new one was too much for her. She was tired at work. She was tired at home. She didn't have any time for herself. After just two months she resigned from her outside work and settled into full-time motherhood.

But it is possible to mesh a career with child care, if you realistically plan. That means, for one thing, getting your child used to the babysitter early on, perhaps even for a day a week from almost the beginning. In that way, they'll be comfortable together and you'll be more relaxed as well. The more confident you are that your baby is in good hands, the less guilt you'll feel at leaving. Managing both a career and child care also means having a backup babysitter, or other arrangement, in case the caretaker you've employed is unavailable for a day or more. And it means, ideally, having a mate who is willing to share the responsibilities on the home front, putting in some wakeful time at night and some fathering time in the evening. If he's able and willing to take on the daytime shift when the baby or babysitter is ill, so much the better.

To make sure that the time you spend with your child is of high quality, it's a good idea to have a "cooling off" period between career time and mothering time. Too many women rush home from the office into the nursery, changing roles before they've even changed clothes. But that may not be best for you or your child. Says Dr. Gordon, "It's very hard to go from a tension-filled, action-oriented world, where you're gauged and gratified immediately, to a world where the activity and action is on a much lower level, and where you have to adjust to an infant's needs. If you come home exhausted, and don't take the time to decelerate, you can't get to the point where you can enjoy the kind of peace and calm you can know with a child. Your work worries are still with you. And you'll find that you're impatient with yourself and with your child." She suggests trying to cool off physically and emotionally from the day's work, even though this is not always possible. For some women, a shower would be just the thing to relax them; for others, just some time in the easy chair with shoes off and feet up will do the trick. It's a time of transition that will allow you to walk into the nursery calmly, and be the mother you really want to be.

Some women decide, during pregnancy, to take a lengthy hiatus from their careers, but then find themselves less than happy as full-time mothers. They miss their careers, their colleagues. Caring for a baby just isn't totally fulfilling; and if the baby is highly active or colicky, it may be too much. They think back wistfully to the days when they left the house early to do the work they love to do. Although they also love the baby, spending day after day with the baby is another story. It can be a hard adjustment for a career woman who is used to accomplishing a great deal each day, to moving from point A to point B and getting rewarded for it. In caring for a baby, point A is usually the most you can hope for, as you spend day after day on the same chores. All the bottles you wash and diapers you change only bring in their wake more soiled bottles and more dirty diapers. The tasks, though not the most difficult, are repetitive ones, and the rewards, though great, are intangible ones. For some women, these rewards just aren't enough, and they long for the good old days. And so, even if they didn't plan it, they may find themselves back on the job anyway.

Women who are dissatisfied with their initial choices may find themselves making new ones that they hadn't even considered before. Some find themselves a part-time position, a way to "have it all" and come out with one's sanity intact. As we pointed out before, in many ways part-time work is the ideal solution for these early years, satisfying a woman's desires both for career and for parenting. One of Kathryn's patients, a secretary, was able to find a 5:00 P.M. to 9:00 P.M. job doing word processing. In this way, she could spend a lot of time with her new baby, some time out of the house, and very little money for babysitters, as her husband generally stayed with the baby during the evenings. When her child was old enough for nursery school she switched her hours to the mornings so she and her husband could share more time together.

Other women find that this is the perfect time to go in a new career direction, particularly one that allows them to work from the home. And so they start up a home business, or a writing career, or anything else that their imagination and talent suggest to them. In that way they stretch themselves in new directions, and don't miss out on being with their children. Many of Kathryn's patients with secretarial experience take on typing jobs at home, once they become mothers. In that way they can both keep up their skills and keep an eye on the baby. Naomi was a former nursery school teacher and the wife of a graduate student. The family's financial situation dictated that she earn money, yet she didn't want to leave the baby. Her solution was to babysit for other people's children in her own home. Her baby had built-in playmates, she had the continuing challenge of working with young children, and she was earning the money the family needed.

Returning to school on a part-time basis is yet another option that some mothers of young children choose. These mothers have plenty of time to spend with their children, yet at the same time they are preparing themselves for their own exciting futures. Having a baby does *not* spell the end of your future as a working woman. It is the beginning of a new future for you and for your family, and you may be very surprised at where it leads you.

11

Preparation, Labor, and Delivery: The Birth of Your Baby

Pregnancy is in itself a consuming experience, but it is really just a transitional stage in a woman's life, a stage of preparation for the birth of a child. As soon as a woman learns she is pregnant, she marks on her calendar the date that pregnancy is expected to give way to motherhood. Becoming a mother is what pregnancy is all about; giving birth is the culmination. Toward the end of pregnancy more and more thought is given to that moment. As the due date approaches, the birth experience seems more real, and concerns about it become more pressing.

One common concern among pregnant women involves just how accurate that due date is. Will the baby really be born on that exact date? Or will it fight its way out sooner, or perhaps nestle longer in the warmth of its mother's body? A due date is most likely to be close to target if a woman recalls the exact date that her last menstrual period began. The doctor uses that date as a guide to predicting the baby's arrival. (The length of a woman's menstrual cycle will also affect the predicted date of birth; be sure to tell your physician if your cycle is longer or shorter than the typical twenty-eight days.) But even if a woman's memory is calendar-perfect, and her cycle as predictable as the monthly rebirth of the moon, the due date is no more than an estimate. While most babies are delivered within two weeks before or after their predicted arrival, the chances are great that your baby's due date will *not* be your baby's birth date.

Taking Its Time

One of the most psychologically trying aspects of a pregnancy is the waiting—especially past your due date. The crib is ready to be slept in. The baby blanket is waiting to be cuddled in. And the telephone is ringing off the hook with queries of why you're still there to answer it. An unexpected delay in the birth date can be especially hard for women who are used to being in control. They can plan most of the important things in their life—but apparently not this event. And as the days pass, they feel the tension of the wait.

Approximately 15% of first-time mothers are at least two weeks overdue in giving birth. The potential problems from the delay are more than psychological. Medically, the baby may be harmed by too long a delay. The placenta actually ceases to function properly when it gets too old, perhaps because of vascular changes. And the baby's increasing size may make demands on the placenta that are simply too great to be adequately met. The baby may consequently be born malnourished, or susceptible to lung trouble, or even stillborn. To avoid these problems, many medical centers give women nonstress tests (described in chapter 6) starting a week or so after the due date to see if the baby is in trouble. If the baby is two or more weeks overdue, labor may be artificially induced to further ensure a healthy baby.

A less common but even riskier situation occurs when a baby is born too soon. Government statistics indicate that about one out of twenty first-born babies are born more than a month ahead of schedule. The reasons for this include multiple birth, an abnormally shaped uterus or cervix, a weakness in the cervix, an overly large baby, or an infection leading to early rupture of the membranes. If the baby is less than a month early, there is generally no problem. In all likelihood it will be completely healthy. But if the birth occurs sooner than that, medical problems may proliferate, such as chronic lung problems, brain damage, cerebral palsy, and seizures.

Prematurity is the number one cause of infant mortality. Even when the baby survives, it may face potential complications. Techniques are now being developed to forestall dangerously early delivery. (Currently, medication is used to stop premature contractions. This treatment is successful in a high percentage of cases.) The aim is to keep babies in long enough—but not too long.

Some of Kathryn's earliest obstetrical experiences involved premature infants; she spent the first four months of her internship working in a premature intensive care unit. Since that time, ten years ago, she's seen dramatic advances in the care of "preemies," as well as in their survival rate. There is better monitoring possible now, improved medication available, more sophisticated diagnostic capabilities and, most important, more research and more experience in this area. Even so, prematurity is one of the most frightening birth complications because a baby who *would* have been perfectly normal instead faces potentially serious complications. It is worth doing everything possible to prevent prematurity. In most cases, the baby's best incubator is its mother.

The Beginning of the End

However realistic or unrealistic the due date turns out to be, women approaching it will begin to experience fairly predictable changes. These occur as the body is preparing to give birth and the baby preparing to be born. Some of them were mentioned earlier in the book, such as increasing insomnia, and urination, and swelling, and general discomfort. As the bones in the pubic area separate, and the joints relax, you become wobblier than ever. Standing up becomes a difficult business, and even walking is a great challenge. As the baby moves down it may cause pressure on the sciatic nerve, leading to back pain and leg pain.

But as the baby's head drops into the pelvis there may be a rather pleasant sensation that goes along with it—a sensation known as "lightening." Occurring usually during a first pregnancy, it takes the pressure off a woman's chest area and makes her breathing easier. (In a second or subsequent pregnancy the abdominal wall is generally so lax that the baby will move forward, instead of down, for the extra room it needs as it grows and gets ready for birth.)

A very different sensation that you may have felt throughout most of your pregnancy commonly intensifies during the last two or three months before the birth. Known as Braxton-Hicks contractions, they involve a cramping and tightening of the uterus. Some women may confuse Braxton-Hicks contractions with the onset of labor, but there are more differences than similarities. They produce hardening of the uterus, as do labor contractions, but they may last longer, and their strength remains about the same from contraction to contraction, without the escalation characteristic of labor pain. The most telling difference is that Braxton-Hicks contractions are not painful. But they are not useless, either. They prime the uterus for delivery by beginning to soften up the cervix. They also give the woman a very mild introduction to the sensation of a uterine contraction, a sensation that she will experience at much fuller force during the actual labor process.

During the last few days or weeks of the pregnancy another change may occur that sends some women to the hospital maternity wing, but really shouldn't. The mucous plug of the cervix may become dislodged. This white or clear plug generally comes out with a small amount of blood, and so may take on a pinkish hue or have streaks of blood in it. Its emergence does *not* mean that labor is necessarily imminent unless other, more telling symptoms are also present. Nor does it mean that an infection is active or brewing. What it does mean is that the cervix is dilated to a certain point—perhaps one and a half or two centimeters—allowing the mucous plug to loosen and fall away. That is a sign that the pregnancy is progressing toward its inevitable conclusion, not that a mad dash to the hospital is in order.

Trips to the hospital are not called for without clear symptoms of labor or of a serious medical complication, but frequent visits to the doctor's office are. Toward the end of pregnancy your doctor will give you a new schedule of office visits involving more frequent, and more thorough, examinations. Internal examinations are generally done at this time to check out the healthy progress of the pregnancy and to uncover any existing or developing problems. It's a good sign if your baby is head down at this advanced stage of pregnancy; the baby is so relatively large by this time that there is little room for it to maneuver around into a breech position. If the head is already "engaged," or firmly fixed in the pelvis, the doctor may tell you to have your bag ready, just in case. Engagement is a sign, though not a guarantee, that labor will not be very long in coming. For a woman expecting a second or subsequent baby, engagement may not occur until labor has already begun.

One of the major things that the doctor will be checking out during these internal examinations is the condition of the cervix. How soft and how thinned out (effaced) is it? And how far has it dilated? During labor the cervical opening will widen to ten centimeters—approximately four inches—but dilation to two or three centimeters can occur even before labor begins. It is one more part of the pattern that leads to the eventual birth, and one more guide, though not an infallible one, to when the birth will occur. Again, the pattern is somewhat different in a woman who has given birth before. Her cervix may well be effaced before the last weeks of pregnancy, and dilation will proceed more easily and more rapidly.

Gaining Knowledge, Fighting Fear

The body's final preparations for delivery are an exciting indication of the labor and the birth that lie ahead; they are also an indication that you and your husband should be doing a different kind of preparing. You should be readying yourselves, intellectually and psychologically, for the birth experience and for what comes after. Pregnancy is prime time for reading books on the pregnancy itself, the delivery, and infant care. It is also a good time for talking to couples who are or who have been in the same situation. What you read and hear can be most helpful if you filter it intelligently to come out with what's valuable and makes sense for you. Someone else's experience won't be exactly the same as yours, but it can add to your fund of knowledge about the process of birth, making it seem both less mysterious and less frightening.

Another aspect of preparation, touring the place where you will give birth, is something you may have done earlier in your pregnancy. If you haven't, it's still not too late. In some ways, this is the best time of all, when you are more informed about the questions you should be asking, more alert to what you should be looking for, more attuned to the reality that you will actually be making use of these facilities, that your baby will be born right here, and that it won't be very long now.

When most people think of preparation they think of classes designed to get parents ready for the childbirth experience. These childbirth preparation classes are an excellent way of getting ready for the big event. Originally they were referred to as "natural childbirth" classes; their aim, presumably, was to prepare mothers for a drug-free labor and delivery and for minimal medical intervention in the birth process. While the role of medications was generally discussed, participants often came away with the message that they had better get by without them. So even if labor turned out to be especially long and difficult, women attempted to agonize their way through it; if they finally succumbed to chemical pain relief, it was with a feeling of failure—that they weren't brave enough to make it.

To combat such feelings, many childbirth educators have expanded the scope of their instruction, emphasizing that their classes are for "prepared childbirth," not necessarily "natural childbirth." The idea currently in favor is to understand the birth process, to learn to remain in control of the pain, but at the same time to learn when external pain relief is warranted both for the good of the mother and the progress of the labor. More mature mothers often find it easier than women in their twenties to accept this premise and to bend the rules a bit for a "natural" birth. They tend to be more realistic about their own capacities, perhaps less doctrinaire and idealistic than their younger counterparts, and even more eager for the type of control that some anesthetic agents seem to impart.

Even the mates of these mature mothers may find the newer, less rigid approach more to their liking. One father who was in a perfect position to compare—with children born seven years apart—was much happier with Lamaze the second time around. "When Gregory was born, in 1976, Lamaze had an air of mysticism about it. I likened it to mutual hypnosis. We all came to believe that labor wouldn't hurt. A woman couldn't even admit she felt pain, much less take something for it. That set up a lot of people for disappointment and for feelings of inadequacy. This time the approach was much more even-handed. The stress was on knowing the facts and on understanding the role of medication, not on damning it."

Some women approach the birth of a baby with a very different idea than "natural" in mind. They don't want to know about pain. They don't want to know about panting and pushing. They want to be basically out of it, preferably unconscious, until after the baby is born. So what's the point of attending a class if you're sure that "natural" is not for you, and that even "prepared" is out of your league? For one thing, you can gain valuable information from the parts of the class not directly related to childbirth. Many classes are broadening their scope to cover such topics as nutrition, exercise, and child care. Some classes begin earlier in pregnancy, and discuss all the problems that can come up in normal and complicated pregnancies. Both the physical and emotional needs of women at various stages of pregnancy are addressed. At whatever stage of pregnancy preparation begins, it provides you with the support and encouragement of people in a like situation. It's comforting to know that other women are having the same feelings and similar problems; it's instructive to find out how other people handle the many challenges of expectant parenthood. The "group" aspect of the class commonly continues even after all members of the group have given birth. Often preparation class reunions are held, and include the newest members of the group—the babies. In addition, countless rewarding friendships have begun between parents at this similar stage of their childbearing careers. But aside from these important extras, even the actual childbirth part of the class can serve a "reluctant" mother well. Although she started out as a disbeliever, she may be lucky enough to have a short and relatively easy labor. By using the breathing and relaxation techniques learned in class and practiced at home, she may be able to get through the birth with little or no medication, and little or no pain.

One of Kathryn's patients who went reluctantly to Lamaze class focused mostly on the explanations of the anesthetic agents. She decided that an epidural was for her, and that she would not be a martyr. As it turned out, she didn't have to be. When she came to the hospital she was already eight centimeters dilated, too close to delivery to be given an epidural. She made it through the labor and birth with very little pain. She had never meant to go "natural," but her classes, and the workings of her body, had made it possible.

Despite their additional attractions, the crux of these classes involves gaining an understanding of the childbirth process, and learning how to remain in control with the minimal amount of drugs needed in your particular case. You'll learn, stage by stage, what to expect, what will be happening to your body and to your baby, what the contractions will be like, when the peaks of pain will come.

You can't be taught how *much* pain you'll feel—that's a completely individual matter. Some women find the pain to be mild and quite bearable, others consider it moderate, while still others report such excruciating pain that they can't imagine ever going through another birth (though with time the memory of the pain dulls enough to allow them to change their minds). One woman compares what she went through to an athletic endeavor: "To me it was like running a marathon. It was as if somebody made me run twenty-six miles with a whip at my back. I was ready to pass out, I ached all over, my chest hurt, my back hurt, but they made me keep going. That's what it seemed like to me." Despite the difficulty, she was willing to go through it again. Her second labor, with a twin pregnancy, was different: "I had a very short labor with the twins, only two hours. But it was two hours of intense, severe pain. It was a searing, ripping-you-apart kind of pain. The positive part was that it was much easier to push out the twins than it had been to push out my son. It was just one quick push for each."

Many factors operate to determine the level of pain a laboring woman feels. They include the size of the baby, its position, and the size and shape of the woman's pelvis. Another important factor, however, is the woman's level of anxiety. A highly anxious woman will tense her muscles, slowing down labor's progress. Her fright will make the whole experience seem worse than it is, and the pain will magnify in her mind as well as in her body until it reaches an unbearable pitch. Anxiety is a result of facing the unknown; an attitude of relative calm is a result of learning just what that unknown will bring. And that's where preparation classes come in. By arming their students with the facts, they are arming them against overwhelming anxiety. They are teaching them that labor is something to be faced, not to be fought.

Childbirth preparation classes also provide direct methods of pain management. Lamaze, for example, the most popular form of childbirth preparation in this country, teaches a set pattern of relaxation and breathing techniques. The idea is for the woman to focus on something other than the contraction so that her perception of it as painful is minimized. With daily practice at home, she will be conditioned to begin the Lamaze routine at the start of each contraction. She will be in control of the labor as the labor builds, not at the mercy of a crescendo of pain.

The Bradley method of childbirth education, most popular in the western states, is an alternative based on training in progressive relaxation. The woman is trained to recognize any tension building in various muscle groups throughout her body, and to release the tension at will. As the proponents of this method assert, the woman is learning to cooperate with her body, rather than to undermine its natural functioning.

Whatever the particular method of pain management used, all share the goal of putting you in control of what is happening to you. You become an active agent, not a passive victim, and feel the rewards of labor even as you're experiencing it. Some women begin to relish this feeling of control even before labor, as they learn and practice the technique they will be using. "Preparation was very important to me because it began to put me in control of the delivery," recalls one mother of her Lamaze classes. "Finally, I was able to do something concrete to assist this child in life. The participation of my husband was also very important. It meant that I wasn't so dependent on my obstetrician. I could depend on my husband to support me from the beginning. By preparing together we began to develop a working relationship in regard to this child. That's proven to be very valuable."

The involvement of the father is one of the great advances—and advantages—of the childbirth education movement. It has marked a sharp departure from past practices, in which the father was relegated to nervous pacing before the delivery and nervous pride after it. Now it is becoming more the norm for the father to be included in the entire process, coaching and supporting his wife during the labor, watching the delivery, holding his newborn baby. What's made this possible is the preparation he's received as part of the childbirth education program. Fathers as well as mothers are taught the physical facts about labor and birth and the appropriate techniques for pain relief. Often, in class, expectant fathers are encouraged to try out the techniques themselves to gain a clearer understanding of what their wives will be doing and what *they* should be doing to help out. Their participation is rewarding for them and for their wives. It enhances a woman's confidence to know that she will not be going through the birth all alone, that someone who has a deep personal interest in it will be there to encourage and support her, that the baby will be welcomed into the world by both its parents. Research has shown that a father's active participation in delivery enhances the quality of the experience both for him and for his wife. Childbirth education and participation are definitely not for women only.

Childbirth education has recently expanded even beyond the husband-wife couple. There are now groups oriented toward single parents, who often use friends or family members as coaches; there are special classes designed to prepare the siblings of the new baby for the birth and its aftermath; there are even some courses designed to help grandparents understand what their role will be as a new generation is added to their family.

As class offerings proliferate, and as your pregnancy progresses from its middle months to its last months, you may wonder exactly how to go about finding the right class for you and when to do it. It's best to start the typical six-week preparation course about two months before your due date (not much earlier or your skills may grow rusty; not much later or your baby may not wait until you've graduated). One good way to locate a class is through your doctor's recommendation; another way is by writing to The International Childbirth Education Association, Inc., P.O. Box 248, Minneapolis, Minnesota 55420, for the location of groups in your area; that organization will forward your request to a state coordinator, who will send you the information. Some preparation classes are located in hospitals and offer definite advantages to the women who will give birth there. The instructors can apprise their students of the specific routines and practices of that particular institution, reducing even further the element of the unknown. But some private preparation groups tell potential clients that they will offer a more consumer-oriented approach, suggesting what hospital practices should be questioned, emphasizing the woman's rights as a patient. Independent of the hospital, their attitude toward traditional hospital procedures is often more critical. Whether a hospital class or private class is right for you is a decision that only you can make, based on your needs and preferences, as well as class location and availability.

There is yet another type of preparation class offered to pregnant women in many areas. It centers not on the birth itself but on feeding the baby after it is born. As increasing numbers of women choose to breast-feed, they want to know what they should be doing during pregnancy to get themselves and their breasts ready for this very new experience. Through classes and specialized books on breast-feeding, as well as through talks with breast-feeding friends, they can learn just what to expect, and what to do to enhance the experience for themselves and their babies. Some of the classes provide a live "model"; for many women, it is the first real-life exposure they've ever had to breast-feeding.

Another part of the preparation involves teaching the women how to prepare their nipples for the baby's suckling. The basic idea is to toughen them up through techniques such as rubbing them with a rough towel, rolling them between thumb and fore-finger, having one's mate stimulate them manually and orally. If the nipples are made less tender during the last months of pregnancy, they will be less sensitive to the baby's often vigorous sucking, and breast-feeding will be more likely to succeed. Such preparation is most important for fair-skinned, fair-haired women because of their special skin sensitivity. There are additional tech-niques described in classes and in books for women who have inverted nipples—those that retract rather than protrude. With a little advance planning, those women can find breast-feeding as satisfactory—and satisfying—as can anyone else.

For those women who plan to bottle-feed, there are also classes available. While there is less physical preparation involved—aside from stocking up with the right supplies—you may feel you need psychological support for your choice of a "less accepted" option. Some women feel ostracized for their decision, less "motherly" for wanting to use bottle instead of breast. But bottle-feeding can be both nutritionally adequate and emotionally satisfying for the infant, and an important component of a strong mother-infant bond. A woman who is confident in her decision can prepare herself for any criticism she may face as she gets ready to care for her baby in a way that is comfortable for her and right for her family.

Doctors on Call

During these last months of your pregnancy, there are two other people whose help you can elicit in preparing for childbirth and for your child. One is someone you may not have even met yet— your pediatrician. If you already have a child, you most likely have a pediatrician. This is the time to go over with him or her all your questions about the earliest days of childhood, questions about your pediatrician's role at the hospital, about feeding decisions and regimens, about signs of potential problems, about the schedule of visits and vaccinations after the birth. Again the idea is to know ahead of time what you can expect, and what may *not* go exactly according to expectations. Even if you remember well how it went last time, it's a good idea to get an update from your doctor. Medical beliefs and practices frequently shift even in a relatively short period of time, and you should be familiar with any changes relevant to your newest child.

For first-time mothers, the only pediatrician they may know is the hometown doctor who treated them as a child. In most cases it's time to find a new one, and now is as good a time as any. "Interviewing" the pediatrician has become an increasingly popular part of prenatal preparation, as many pregnant women want to select this important person in their baby's life even before the baby is born. Through recommendations of friends and of physicians they make appointments to speak with various pediatricians (or with family practitioners who treat both children and adults), and ask them questions about philosophical approach and actual practice. This is definitely a positive development, as long as it's not overdone. It probably is not necessary to interview every doctor in town before winnowing them down to the one you like best. If you find one physician in whom you feel confident, and whose medical views and nutritional beliefs make sense to you, you may want to save your strength and stop the search, trusting your judgment unless the doctor later gives you reason to doubt it. If the first doctor you interview seems to suit you, there's no pressing reason to look further. Just as with an obstetrician, an advance interview provides quite limited information. Only when you see the pediatrician in action with your child will you know whether you have made the right choice.

The other doctor who will be instrumental in your preparation is your obstetrician, providing assistance that goes far beyond the medical exam described earlier. As your due date approaches, there are many issues you'll want to discuss that you may not have touched on earlier in your pregnancy or at your initial interview. The following are some common—and important—questions you may want to ask: At what signs of labor should I call you? What are the procedures once I arrive at the hospital? Do they include shaving and an enema? Will I be routinely placed on a fetal monitor? Will I be able to walk around in early labor? Will you be at the hospital all through the labor or, if not, at what point will you arrive? Will my husband be allowed to be present during labor and delivery? Are there any situations in which he would not be allowed to be with me? Will the family have time together after the baby is born, or will the baby be taken away immediately?

Making a Difference

The major reason to ask such questions is to find out what will confront you. The more you know, the less there is to fear. But there is also another reason. On some issues your views may have an influence on just what your experience will be. If you have good lines of communication with your doctor, and are able to explain convincingly why you want something done a certain way, you may be able to strike a compromise or even accomplish a change in a particular policy for your case.

"Prepping" is one procedure that is often susceptible to change. The practice of shaving is not as popular now as it once was, and if you object to it, your physician may agree to forego it. Some women shave off all their pubic hair at home once labor begins because they would rather do it themselves. Many physicians require only that the hair be shaved off in the area where the episiotomy will be done, or not at all.

The other part of the "prep," the enema, is still quite prevalent, and your doctor may or may not let you labor without one. The basic idea of the enema is to clear out the fecal material from the lower bowel so that it won't be expelled on the delivery table during the birth. Some doctors believe that an enema will also stimulate labor and make it more comfortable. But more doctors are now leaving the decision up to the patient, so it's worth your advance consideration. If you think that you wouldn't be embarrassed defecating with other people watching, you may prefer to avoid the artificial stimulation of an enema. An enema taken at home at the beginning of labor may serve a similar function to the hospital enema, satisfying both your needs and any objections that your doctor may have. But whatever your preferences regarding the "prep," it's a good idea to discuss it with your doctor at this stage.

Another common procedure under increasing question is the

episiotomy. Many women are asking that their doctors not do it unless it is absolutely medically necessary, and many doctors are following those instructions, allowing the mother more control over her childbirth experience. An episiotomy, a surgical cut in the perineum (the area between the vagina and the rectum), is done for two basic reasons. One involves a question of medical urgency: The baby's heartbeat is decreasing, and the delivery process must be speeded up. In these cases an episiotomy will hasten the end of labor and help prevent serious oxygen deprivation to the baby. The other rationale involves the elasticity of the mother's perineal tissues. There is clinical evidence, though it has not been scientifically tested or proved, that some women who have spent a long time pushing an average-sized or large baby through the vagina without an episiotomy will experience stretching and tearing of muscle fibers in the perineum. These are microscopic rips, not the jagged tears often spoken of and written about. Such tiny rips are thought to be related to a prolonged pushing stage, and may eventually lead to reduced bladder control or prolapse of the uterus, bladder, or rectum. This may require surgical repair at a later time.

If there is no threat to the baby, many women would prefer not to undergo an episiotomy and the discomfort that follows it. The negative side of an episiotomy *is* the discomfort, which can last up to a month after the birth and is especially intense during intercourse. It can last even longer than a month in breast-feeding mothers, whose vaginas generally do not lubricate well. If you have doubts about the episiotomy, discuss it with your doctor. He or she may agree not to do an episiotomy unless it is medically indicated for the good of the child. But the final decision cannot be made until near the end of labor. If you feel that an episiotomy is right for you, give your doctor the go-ahead. The important thing, whatever your preference, is to understand what's involved ahead of time, to be open to your doctor's views, and to be comfortable with your final decision.

The Anesthetic Arsenal

One of the most important issues to discuss with your doctor during the weeks before your due date, even if you've gone over it before, is that of pain-relieving medication. Most likely you will have at least some control over this aspect of the birth, and your knowledge of the available options will help you to make intelligent choices.

You may be approaching this subject from one of three perspectives. The first is that you don't want to read it. You have absolutely no intention of taking any medications for pain, so why waste your time learning about them? The problem with that stance is that even the best of intentions can go awry. As we mentioned earlier, a long and difficult labor may necessitate intervention, including drugs, and taking them does not signal failure. A woman who tenses up her muscles due to stress and pain will hold the baby in, slowing up its delivery. Taking some medication may relax her enough to allow her to cooperate with the labor process. And it may make labor a more positive experience.

At the other end of the spectrum are women who feel that medication is inevitable because they won't be able to bear the pain, especially at their age. Won't the labor be so complicated and so agonizing that anesthesia—or at least analgesia—is mandatory? Not necessarily. In fact, a recent study of 75 mothers from the Washington metropolitan area, who ranged in age from 38 to 49, revealed that 58% of them gave birth without any kind of medication. The point is that you can't anticipate the kind of labor you'll have. You can't know for sure how short or long, or easy or hard, your labor will be. If you're the third kind of woman, the one who approaches this subject with an open mind, then you'll approach your labor with a firm grasp of the facts about medication, and the wherewithal to use those facts to the best advantage for you and your baby.

There are two basic types of pain medication used for childbirth. One is the analgesics, which are given in either small amounts intravenously or larger amounts intramuscularly to provide their pain-relieving effects. They act, essentially, by reducing the ability of nerves to transmit pain, and produce some drowsiness or even a dreamy state in the mother. One common criticism is that they also cause sluggishness in the baby, and perhaps even depress its respiration. But if given at the proper times and in the proper amounts, these narcotic agents (such as Demerol and morphine) appear to have minimal effects on a mature baby. Although there are many available analgesic agents, most hospitals have only two or three of them in their drug armamentarium for childbirth. Many women can make it through labor without using anything else, except for a local anesthetic at the delivery. Even if they also find that they need more anesthetic, later, the dosage requirement may be less because of the analgesic's effects.

When many women think of that other type of pain medication for childbirth—the anesthetics—they visualize a woman lying helpless and unconscious as her baby is taken from her. That is still the case in some instances, but not many. General anesthesia was for quite a long time the preferred method of pain relief for childbirth. Just a whiff of chloroform or ether, and pain and consciousness were both soon blotted out. But in recent decades that so-called advantage has turned into a disadvantage. Women for the most part *want* to witness their babies being born, if not to feel it, at least to see it, if not to fully participate, at least to observe. They *want* to have the experience, and the memory, of that most special moment. There are also medical disadvantages that are reducing the use of general anesthesia for childbirth. While the mother is unconscious, some of her stomach contents may be regurgitated and may become lodged in her lungs. Pneumonia, and maternal mortality, may result. The baby may also be adversely affected by the anesthesia, and born in a physically depressed state. Because of such serious potential side effects, general anesthesia is rarely used for vaginal deliveries today. One exception is in the case of fetal distress requiring a quick forceps delivery. In that situation a general anesthetic may be used because it is the quickest and most effective agent.

What has widely replaced general anesthesia in recent years are regional anesthetics—agents that block the nerves that carry pain signals from the pelvic area to the brain. The woman is "numbed" in the area that counts, but left awake and alert to follow her doctor's instructions as well as to witness her baby's birth. Another advantage is that these anesthetics are believed to have little direct effect on the baby. In fact, they are sometimes touted as "ideal" anesthetics for childbirth, but as we shall see, they do have drawbacks.

A very popular type of regional anesthetic is the epidural, which involves injecting small doses of an anesthetic drug (similar to Novocain used in dentistry) into the canal surrounding the spinal cord through a plastic tube. That tube can be left in place for hours, and additional anesthetic added to it to keep the numbness from wearing off. The anesthetic blocks the nerves as they leave the spinal cord. Another option is a caudal, which is similar to an epidural, except that it is introduced at the very tip of the spine. Either an epidural or caudal can be initiated fairly early in labor, protecting the woman from the worst of the pain, turning a potentially agonizing experience into a pain-free interlude of expectancy and excitement. But sometimes it doesn't work out so well. The anesthesiologist must be skilled to correctly administer an epidural or caudal, and many hospitals are not equipped for the demands of the procedure. As a result, this form of anesthesia is not offered at every facility. Even with a skilled anesthesiologist, the medication takes some time to take effect, and may produce "spotty" results, with the pelvic area not sufficiently numb. Sometimes the tube is not located in the proper location, and then must be reinserted. Another possible problem is that the anesthetic may cause the mother's blood pressure to drop, which in turn could produce a reduction in the baby's heartbeat.

Probably the biggest drawback to epidurals and caudals is that they can interfere with the process of labor. That can happen in two ways. They may slow down the uterine contractions to such a degree that a chemical must be administered to stimulate good, productive labor to continue. Also, they inhibit the woman's ability to push out the baby. She does not feel the instinctive urge to push, so she must do it by following the nurse's instructions, not her body's. More women who have epidurals during labor end up having a forceps delivery than do those who forego the epidural. One way of reducing this disadvantage is to let the anesthesia wear off toward the end of labor; in that way, the woman will be sensitive to her body's signals in time to do effective pushing. But it is not an easy thing to subject oneself to pain after hours of relief, and few women choose to do so.

Another form of regional anesthetic is the spinal, or "saddle block." Involving an injection of an anesthetic drug into the spinal canal, it effectively numbs the woman from the waist down. The disadvantage of this technique is that because of its marked slowing effect on the labor it cannot be administered until shortly before delivery. The woman has already suffered the worst, going through the pains of the most severe contractions, so why subject herself to powerful medication so near the end of the labor process? For this very short period of relief, she may find herself suffering from a spinal headache—a severe, long-lasting pain that sometimes follows spinal taps or spinal anesthesia—or other complications.

There are other, more sensible methods of pain relief which can be used at the time of delivery. One is a simple local anesthetic—the injection of a pain-relieving medication such as Novocain in the area of the vagina. Such drugs have no effect on the baby, and they wear off very soon after the delivery. Another choice at this point is a pudendal block. An injection of local anesthetic with a long needle can be inserted through the vagina to block the nerves that come down to the perineum. Its numbing action takes effect quickly, and is potent enough to allow for an episiotomy or a forceps delivery.

As you can see, the question of "natural" versus "medicated" childbirth is not an all-or-none proposition. There are many different levels and types of pain relief, and you should have some familiarity with all of them. Actually, you may be able to simplify your learning task a bit by finding out ahead of time just what analgesic agents are used at the center where you'll be delivering. That's one of the questions you should ask your physician toward the end of your pregnancy. You should also find out what your doctor's preferences in medication are ahead of time; when you are in labor, you may not be prepared to engage in a rational discussion about the pros and cons of the various agents. Another issue to address in your doctor's office is just how the medication decision is made once labor begins. Are *you* expected to make the request for a pain-relieving drug, or will the doctor evaluate the situation and recommend, or order, that the medication be given? It's important that you know how this works ahead of time so you won't be surprised, perhaps unpleasantly, by the procedure during labor. To take medication is not necessarily to give up control of the birth; to remain ignorant of the biological and medical process is.

Induction of Labor: the Right Time, the Right Reason

You will also want to bring up another issue to your doctor as your pregnancy nears its end: Should you or shouldn't you have your labor artificially induced? If induction is necessary, it is generally done by the administration of oxytocin (trade-named Pitocin), a hormone produced in the pituitary gland. Oxytocin is a very potent substance that generally causes the uterus to begin contracting within half an hour. It is usually given intravenously; a patient must be closely monitored while the drug is administered and exerting its effects. Some hospitals are experimenting with the use of prostaglandins—a substance that also produces uterine contractions—to induce labor. Another method sometimes used involves puncturing the amniotic sac to rupture the membranes. For women who have been through childbirth before, and who are already dilated three or four centimeters, that may be all that's required to initiate the labor process.

Elective inductions are quite common in Europe, but have become less acceptable here. In fact, the American College of Obstetricians and Gynecologists has taken a position against induction being done for the sake of patient or doctor convenience; only when medical reasons for it exist should labor be induced. There are a number of situations in which the induction of labor is medically indicated (see chapter 6). For example, if the mother is a diabetic or a hypertensive, and tests indicate that the baby is under stress because of her condition, labor may be induced to avoid serious damage to the child. An overly long pregnancy is another reason to remove the baby from an increasingly hostile environment. If the woman's membranes rupture prematurely—an event that occurs in about 15% of pregnancies—labor will be induced unless it begins spontaneously within twelve hours or so. It's important that the baby's birth not be unduly delayed after the rupture of membranes to prevent the development of a potentially dangerous infection. Still another reason for induction, which might seem on the surface to be elective, really does have a sound medical basis. Say that a woman has a history of fast labors, is five centimeters dilated and full term, and lives an hour from the hospital. To prevent a "taxicab" birth, the doctor may decide to induce the labor instead of waiting for a frantic phone call. Given that a hospital is a safer place to deliver than is the back seat of a cab, the woman and her baby would be medically better off for that decision.

The decision to induce labor should not be made lightly, because the procedure does have certain potential drawbacks. For one thing, it may not work well if the woman is not physically ready for it. To be a good candidate, the woman should be at or very close to term, the baby's head should be engaged, and the cervix should be effaced and softened. If those conditions don't exist, induction may go on for twenty-four hours or more with little effect, and a Cesarean delivery may be the result. So the woman who opted for the "convenience" of induction may end up with more than a little inconvenience.

Although an induction generally produces a labor that is shorter than the average, it can also produce a harder one. What happens is that the very early part of labor, when things are going slowly and little pain is felt, is often skipped over, and strong labor takes hold quickly. Without a gradual buildup the woman may be unprepared for the strength of the contractions. If the oxytocin is not administered properly—in a gradually increasing fashion—the contractions may not only be strong but very close together, with little or no time to relax between them. Such painful, unrelenting contractions can be very difficult for the mother to bear as well as stressful for some babies. But that problem can be largely avoided through the use of monitors that register the strength of uterine contractions. The doctor can adjust the dosage of oxytocin accordingly, lowering it or even stopping it for a time if the contractions are too frequent and forceful. Induction of labor, if done for the right reasons and in the right way, can be an invaluable tool in preventing fetal damage. But if used indiscriminately and done improperly, it can make matters worse for both the mother and the baby. If you are well versed in both the benefits and drawbacks of induction, you can make sure that it's used only to your advantage.

Countdown to Birth

Once you've armed yourself with information about the labor and delivery process, you may find that the hardest part is waiting for the labor to begin. You may even worry that you won't recognize labor when it happens to you, or that you may mistake some gas pains for the real thing. Some women do go through what's known as "false labor," and find themselves making several round trips to the hospital. These false labor pains (which may be different from Braxton-Hicks contractions) are tricky because they are painful, sometimes even more painful than true labor. But they differ from labor in that they don't help the cervix to dilate or the baby to descend. In real labor, the uterus contracts from the top all the way down, pushing the baby downward; in false labor, the uterine contractions are disoriented, seemingly random in pattern. If a woman who is experiencing painful contractions finds that they are not increasing in frequency, and that they go away when she stands up or moves around, then they are probably not true labor contractions. But a call to the doctor is in order if there is any doubt.

One of the things you should straighten out with your doctor ahead of time is just when you should call—how fast the contractions should be coming before you alert him or her to your condition. The doctor's advice will probably be based on how far you live from the hospital as well as the length of any previous labor you've had. But contractions may not be your first sign of labor. Another fairly common one, as mentioned earlier, is the rupture of membranes. It may start with a slight leakage or with a sudden gushing of liquid. One woman, whose membranes ruptured while she was sleeping, compared the watery clime of her bed to Niagara Falls. For Joan, it happened right at the start of a World Series game between the Boston Red Sox and the Cincinnati Reds. She had just gotten settled on the couch, with some iced tea and crackers on hand, when the flood began. When her husband called the doctor, he hoped to be told that the trip to the hospital could wait nine innings, but he ended up listening to the game on radio in the labor room. (P.S.: The Reds won, and Joan's older son is an avid baseball fan.)

Some doctors advise their patients to shower rather than to bathe when their due date is near or past; in that way they won't miss this telling passage of fluid. Once the membranes rupture—and even a slight leakage of amniotic fluid is a signal of rupture—your physician should be informed at once. Unless contractions begin soon, induction of labor is a real possibility. There is no reason that labor should be more difficult or dangerous because of ruptured membranes. In fact, physicians often artificially rupture the membranes during labor to speed up the process.

Still another sign of labor is "bloody show," a discharge of blood that can occur when the cervix is thinning out and dilating. Often it happens along with a contraction, and serves as additional confirmation that labor has begun. When bleeding occurs independently of contractions, your doctor should be notified. It may simply be related to cervical dilation, but it can also be the sign of a problem, such as a low placenta, and should be investigated.

If you begin to feel labor pains in the middle of the night, but they are not yet close enough together to warrant a trip to the hospital, it's a good idea to stay in bed and try to get some sleep. If you spend the night awake, in excited anticipation of what's about to happen, you may be very sorry the next night when you're in active labor and exhausted from your prolonged period of wakefulness. But labor that starts slowly, during the day, is best handled by a different strategy. Instead of sitting around and timing your far-apart contractions, go to a movie, or a museum, or anything else that helps take your mind off your body. Soon enough your body will be the focus of all your attention. If you do find yourself passing the time in a movie, try to resist the popcorn. Once labor begins it's best to eat very lightly, mainly clear liquids and semi-solids such as gelatin. Some people vomit during labor, so it's best not to have a full stomach.

Once you reach the hospital, it will seem as if everyone's attention will be on your body. After you've been admitted and have changed your clothes, your blood pressure will be taken, the baby's heartbeat checked, and an internal examination will be conducted. The purpose of the internal exam is to determine the dilation of your cervix and the descent and position of the baby. Internals will be conducted periodically through the labor, by a resident doctor, a labor nurse, or by your own physician. Don't be surprised if they're more painful during labor than they were during your routine office visits. At this time, the nerves to the uterus have sensitized the whole vagina, so the discomfort of the exam will be greater. Later on in labor, the internals may be done during contractions, rather than between them, and may cause even greater discomfort. But the doctor needs the information from this procedure to accurately assess the progress of the labor. Yet another procedure that may be done soon after your hospital admission is the "prepping"—the shaving and the enema—that was discussed earlier. If your doctor agreed to forego those procedures, but is not yet at the hospital to give the order, ask the hospital staff to check your chart for that information.

About an hour or so after your hospital arrival, you'll probably be ready to be wheeled into your birthing or labor room. In some hospitals you'll be hooked up to a fetal monitor at this point and an intravenous infusion will be started. The purpose of the infusion, which is a water and sugar or a water and salt solution, is not primarily to give you energy, as many people believe. Its major function is to provide fluid to prevent dehydration. Dehydration is a real possibility during labor and delivery, especially if the woman is vomiting. An additional, and important, advantage is that an access line is set up for the administration of any other necessary fluids. If an emergency occurs and the laboring woman needs blood, for example, or if labor slows down and oxytocin is necessary to stimulate it, those substances can be administered without delay.

What's going on inside the hospital is complementary to what's going on inside you. You can't help but be aware of profound internal changes, the changes of labor that come in three stages. The first stage is the longest and hardest, lasting about eight to ten hours in a first birth (and about half that in a subsequent birth). It involves the dilation of the cervix to a ten-centimeter opening, which is about the width of a hand. As this stage progresses, the contractions come closer together, last longer, and are more severe. The latter part of this stage is known as transition—a time that few women forget because of the intensity of the pain it brings. Along with the pain may come nausea, chills, shaking, and perspiration, as well as a state of panic. Your training in breathing and relaxation techniques is put to the test now, as is your husband's knowledge and compassion as a coach. This is the time when many of the women who resisted medication earlier decide that they need the relief, that the breathing is just not enough and that relaxation is not attainable under the stress of the pain.

During the first stage of labor, some women find relief by changing their position. They may even be able to walk around for a time before transition starts, depending on whether they're hooked up to fetal monitors and IV's. Some women like to sit up; others position themselves in varying ways in the bed. As long as there is no trouble with the baby's heartbeat, you'll be able to assume any position you're comfortable in during labor. That position will depend both on your individual preference (it's often the one a woman sleeps in) and on whether you're in front or in back labor. If there is a problem with the fetal heartbeat, you will be positioned in a way to improve it, which likely means lying on your left side.

There are various innovations on the market designed to increase the comfort of laboring women. One popular one is the birthing bed, an electric bed that can adjust from a completely sitting up position to a completely flat one, making it easy for the patient to assume different positions. The bottom of the bed can drop off so that the baby can be easily delivered, even if forceps are used. It's as convenient as a delivery table, yet eliminates the need to move the woman during a difficult time in the laboring process. Another innovation, the birthing chair, is really a modernized version of a birthing device that goes back more than 3,000 years. It can be raised, lowered, or tilted, and allows the woman to sit up during both labor and delivery. Although these are interesting additions to the childbirth marketplace, and add to your options, they do not mark revolutionary advances in the field.

While the bed or chair will provide you with the physical support you'll need during labor, you may wonder who will be providing you with the emotional and medical support. Just who will be tending to you during labor? In addition to the person you brought along, your coach, a labor room nurse will play an important role during this time. For one thing, the nurse may also be doing some coaching, as not every husband is as helpful or as competent at this as he'd like to be. While most men do rise to the occasion, some are so distressed at seeing their wives in pain that they discourage the breathing exercises and encourage anesthesia instead.

That's what happened to Anita during labor with her second child. Her first labor had been difficult, and after eight hours she had finally opted for an epidural. This time she hoped to get by with little or no medication. But at the first sign of pain, her husband said to her, "Why go through it again? Forget the breathing and take the medication." With the combination of the labor pain and his pressure, she relented, and again chose an epidural. But the woman who is determined to give Lamaze a go may find herself turning to the nurse for a more optimistic, supportive attitude, and may avoid anesthesia.

Aside from her sometime adjunct coaching role, the nurse will check your blood pressure periodically, and may be administering analgesic medication if you need it. In addition, if you're on a fetal monitor, the nurse will be the person watching it, relaying any important information to you, and changing your position if the monitor reveals a problem with the baby's heartbeat.

If you've noticed that a person of prime importance has not yet been mentioned in this section, that's because that individual may not even be on the scene yet. That person is the doctor. Depending on the number of patients he or she has in labor at the time, and his or her general method of practice, your obstetrician may not arrive at the hospital, or at your bedside, until delivery is imminent. More commonly, doctors check out their patients periodically during labor, and some try to be close by during the entire labor period. This is where midwives excel, as they generally manage to be with their patients throughout this time to reassure them and carefully attend to their health needs. As mentioned earlier, you should find out ahead of time what your doctor's general procedure is and when he or she can be expected to arrive at the scene.

Most physicians are in the hospital by the time the second stage of labor, the expulsion stage, begins. This is the stage that starts with the total dilation of the cervix and ends with the baby's birth. In a first birth, it normally takes anywhere from thirty minutes to two hours; in subsequent births it is generally under an hour in length, and can be as short as five minutes. You'll know it's starting when you feel pressure, as if you're about to have a bowel movement. But you shouldn't follow your urge to push until you get the go-ahead from your doctor or labor nurse. If pushing begins prematurely, before dilation is complete, it can result in a torn or swollen cervix.

Pushing can be a very welcome activity after the long and difficult contractions of transition. This stage brings with it the physical relief of following your body's instincts, as well as the emotional relief of "taking charge" and becoming a more active agent in your baby's birth. "I was glad to reach the point where I could push," said one woman whose first stage of labor lasted ten hours. "Pushing was better than just lying there in cramps. At last I could *do* something to help with the birth." But again, individual differences are important. While some women consider the expulsion stage an absolute breeze compared with what went before, others find it excruciatingly painful, absolutely the worst part of the entire labor.

But as bad as it can sometimes be, at least it signals that labor is nearing an end. During this stage, you will be wheeled into the delivery room, unless the birth is to take place in the labor (or "birthing") room. As you feel the baby moving down the birth canal, and a burning sensation as the baby crowns (its head coming into view at the vulvar opening), your doctor will be getting ready for the delivery, scrubbing up, donning a sterile gown and gloves, applying antiseptic solution to the perineal area. A local anesthetic or pudendal block may be administered at this time and an episiotomy performed. All is now ready for the baby's birth.

In most cases, the birth is the easiest part of the entire labor process. If all is well and the baby is positioned properly, just a few pushes by the mother will enable the doctor to lift the baby's head out. If the position is not the ideal one, however, or the baby is exhibiting signs of distress, forceps may be used to ensure a safe birth. The very word "forceps" conjures up terrible images for some women, images of agony for the mother and deformity for the infant. Those images are based on how things *used* to be, before the advent of Cesarean deliveries. Forceps were employed even if the baby was very high up, a procedure that certainly was both painful and dangerous. But in current medical practice forceps are not used unless the cervix is completely dilated and the baby's head is low in the vagina. The slight pull necessary to get the baby out does not put great force on the baby, or hurt it, or "smash its head," as some people may imagine. A forceps delivery done properly is not likely to cause neurological damage, and no longer deserves a bad reputation.

Whether the baby practically falls out or must be manipulated out by forceps, its birth is a magical moment, all the more magical for parents who have waited so long for it. Whether the labor was swift or arduous, the birth marks its successful completion, a kind of victory over the forces that kept the baby in. For many mothers, crying is a natural response to the birth, tears of joy that the labor is at an end and that the baby is on hand. Remembers one mother of her first childbirth experience, "When I delivered my daughter I let out a cry. It was the most primitive feeling I have ever had of victory, that I produced this person. The feeling was so primitive, it was almost primeval."

Most women expect the joy and the amazement, but are surprised by a reaction of shock. They may be shocked either that they produced something so wonderful, or shocked that their production doesn't seem so wonderful at all. The baby may seem unrecognizable, not at all what they expected, a strange and scrawny little creature who must be someone *else's* baby. That feeling may be heightened if the baby's coloring and features seem very different from one's own. Although Linda Kestenbaum, the New

York psychologist who treats many pregnant women, had her own son more than five years ago, she remembers the feeling well: "I thought my child would have blond hair and a dark complexion because I did. I wanted to see my own image in him. But what came out was a baby with pitch black hair and fair skin. He looked more like my husband than like me. I was shocked. Even after I had held him for an hour I didn't recognize him in the nursery. He didn't fit into my fantasized preconceived notion." For some parents, love takes only a look; for others, it comes after days or weeks or months of caring for this precious, dependent little person. The delay can be disappointing, and the initial reaction of indifference or dismay hard to admit. But it's important to remember that the love *will* come. Although birth marks the end of your pregnancy, it marks a new beginning in the relationship between you and your baby.

After the Birth

The moment of birth may be so emotionally overwhelming that you'll barely even notice the physical part of labor that's drawing to a close. In the next few minutes to half an hour after the birth you'll be delivering something not nearly as interesting as the baby— the placenta, the membranes, and the remainder of the umbilical cord. The contractions that stopped briefly for the birth start up again mildly, and you may be asked to push with them to help expel those uterine contents. There is little or no pain associated with this stage because the birth canal has already been stretched by the baby's descent and emergence. But you may begin to feel very trembly. In fact, many women shake uncontrollably at this time as a result of changing hormone levels. This is something that Joan was totally unprepared for. She had never been told that it might happen, and she thought it was a sign of something seriously amiss. But it is perfectly normal. Joan was expecting to experience it again after her second delivery, but it was milder that time.

Another source of some discomfort may be the uterine massage that is done in many hospitals to help the uterus contract and to prevent excessive bleeding. But something you won't even feel, because of the local or regional anesthetic, will be the sewing up of the episiotomy. Some obstetricians also inspect the cervix and the inside of the vagina after delivery to make sure there's no tearing inside; if there's been any tearing on the inside or the outside, this is the time when the doctor will repair it.

The postbirth procedures vary widely from hospital to hospital. In some centers you'll be allowed to hold your baby right after the birth, to nurse it, and then to spend some time alone as a new family unit—father, mother, baby, and perhaps even older sibling. In others, the baby is whisked away to medical exam and then nursery, you're whisked away to the recovery room or hospitals room, and it may be hours before you meet again. Most hospital do offer a rooming-in arrangement for women who choose it, allowing mother and baby to spend a lot of time together during these first few days. But rooming-in in one hospital may be very different from rooming-in in another, with one permitting the baby much more time out of the nursery. This is something you should inquire about before your hospital stay.

The more liberal the rooming-in policy, the faster and easier the establishment of a good nursing relationship. For mothers who choose to breast-feed, this will be one of the main concerns of these first few days. The maternity nursing staff is generally trained to help you with it, and there may even be a specialist available to assist new nursing mothers who are having difficulty. The main thing to remember is that the first day or two is mainly for practice. The nursing sessions shouldn't be lengthy—just long enough for the baby to get some of the colostrum, and for the two of you to figure out just what you should be doing. Within a few days, your milk will be coming in, your nipples will be tougher, and the breast-feeding sessions can be longer and more productive.

Women who opt not to breast-feed may be expecting to receive medication to dry up their milk supply and to relieve their aching breasts. But some hospitals don't provide such medication because of its side effects, which can include dizziness and nausea. Instead, they either provide breast binders or give instructions on how to devise your own with a sheet or a large towel. Wearing a tight bra is usually not effective in cutting off the milk supply because it's just not tight enough. Such remedies as acetaminophen, aspirin, or ice can all help relieve the pain of milk-filled breasts.

Whether you breast-feed or bottle-feed, you'll have various bodily discomforts to put up with after the baby is born. For one thing, your uterus will be shrinking back to almost its normal size, a process that takes about six weeks. The way it shrinks is through contractions, and as you know by now, contractions can be quite painful. Such afterpains often intensify during nursing. And they are more painful after a second or subsequent birth because the uterus is more out of shape and has more work to do to get down to size. If you've had an episiotomy, you'll also have that discomfort to deal with. What can help is hot showers, as well as perineal exercises, which involve tightening and then relaxing the perineal muscles (something you may have done during your pregnancy).

Constipation is another common postpartum complaint. Although it may sound strange, one of its causes is fear. New mothers are often hesitant to push because it makes them feel as if they're having the baby all over again. And if a woman has had stitches, moving her bowels may make her feel that everything is going to break apart. So a laxative is often prescribed to get her system going again. Once she does have a bowel movement, and she realizes that her body won't fall apart nor a baby fall out, it will be easier for her to go the next time. A related problem is hemorrhoids. Even women who didn't suffer from them before or during the pregnancy may suffer from them now. They are the worst if the pushing stage of labor lasted for a long time. For suggestions on dealing with them, see page 36. No matter what you do for them, they'll probably disappear within two months of the delivery if you didn't have them before the pregnancy.

Many women have trouble urinating for a time after the delivery. Such difficulty is most common in women who spent a long time pushing, who had an epidural, or who didn't urinate during labor and developed an overdistended bladder. If your bladder becomes very overfilled, you may be put on a catheter for a few days to let it contract down to normal size. This problem with urination is most often a temporary one that goes away by itself.

Vaginal bleeding is yet another reality of postpartum life. For about two weeks there is heavy bleeding of bright red blood. After that time the lining of the uterus that supported the placenta liquefies and comes out, creating a reddish-brown strong-smelling discharge.

Fortunately, all those physical annoyances are dwarfed by the emotional aspects of the childbirth experience. Although the elation and euphoria may become laced with feelings of sadness or even depression (as we'll discuss more fully in chapter 13), the sense of satisfaction in having created new life lingers on. It can be most satisfying for women who have had a good dose of life themselves, who have seen what it has to offer, who want to offer it to their children. They can put the pain of childbirth and its aftermath in perspective as they savor the joys of new motherhood.

12

The Cesarean Experience: A Different Kind of Birth

The news can come in different ways, at different times, but it is never news a woman welcomes. She may hear it during a routine office visit, when her doctor discovers that the baby is finally settling into its prebirth position, but settling in feet first. Or she may hear it after she's already been through hours of hard labor, and hours of pushing, and the baby is barely budging, and her efforts seem in vain. The news is that she will be having a Cesarean delivery. All that she has been preparing for, practicing for, hoping for—the experience of a vaginal birth—will not be hers to know, at least not this time.

For the woman who faces it, the news can be shocking, but some people are more shocked by how very often the news is given. Fifteen years ago, just 5% of births were Cesareans; that figure has more than tripled, to 18% in 1981. In some hospitals one in four births is a Cesarean, while in others the rate is nearing one in three. There are some good reasons for the increasing rate of surgical deliveries—and reasons that may be not quite so good. On the positive side, the surgery is safer now because of advances in medical care that include improved anesthetic techniques, more sophisticated blood transfusion capabilities, and the availability of a wider range of antibiotics. As the dangers of Cesareans have declined, so has the use of "high" forceps, a difficult and possibly hazardous procedure that often involved twisting the baby around and pulling it down from way up in the uterus. Cesarean deliveries have undoubtedly saved many lives and prevented the damage that such a difficult forceps delivery could cause. The rise in the number of Cesarean births reflects, in part, a commitment not just to life but to the quality of life. In some cases a Cesarean delivery is the only avenue available for attaining a healthy baby.

Whatever the reasons for the increase in Cesareans, women 35 and over are the most likely to find themselves delivering in this fashion. The Cesarean rate for this age group is one in four and climbing. In 1970, it was only one in twelve. Some of the reasons for a higher rate for older mothers are quite valid, while others are open to question. Older mothers are more likely to suffer from such health problems as high blood pressure and diabetes (see chapter 6), and a Cesarean may be warranted both to ensure their baby's health and to safeguard their own. As a woman gets older, she is also more likely to experience dystocia—a long and painful labor that does not progress normally. Doctors theorize that because her uterus is older its muscle tone is poorer and its contractions not as efficient in pushing the baby out. When labor is apparently not getting the job done, oxytocin is generally administered in an attempt to stimulate productive contractions. But if that doesn't work, and the woman seems still to be laboring in vain, then a Cesarean will be performed to finally achieve the birth of the baby.

Another reason why older mothers are more common candidates for Cesareans involves the doctor's mental attitude rather than the woman's physical condition. Some doctors still consider women over 35 to be high-risk patients, and are afraid that the slightest problem will lead to medical disaster. So if the labor is not the perfect labor, progressing quickly and efficiently, there is a tendency to perform a Cesarean more readily than would be the case with a younger woman. And there is less fear of being criticized for such a decision. After all, this type of thinking goes, the woman is 38, or 40, or 42 . . . certainly the doctor can get the job done better than the patient can. While there is generally little truth in that belief, it is a belief that helps to sustain the higher Cesarean rate for older mothers.

There are other reasons for Cesareans that apply to both younger and older mothers, and all expectant mothers should be aware of them. Cesareans are performed if the woman has an active herpes infection, in order to prevent the baby from being exposed to the virus. They are also done in cases of placenta previa, where the placenta covers the cervical opening, as well as in some cases of fetal distress if the baby is not receiving a sufficient supply of oxygen. The latter may be detected by fetal monitoring or fetal scalp blood sampling, and procedures are immediately instituted to correct it. But if they don't work, and if birth is not imminent, then a Cesarean delivery may be the only way to ensure a healthy baby.

One of the most common reasons for a Cesarean birth is termed cephalopelvic disproportion—in simpler terms, the mother's pelvis is not large enough for the baby to fit through. Push as she may, the baby isn't going anywhere. Sometimes this problem is suspected even early in pregnancy when the doctor discovers, through clinical examination, that a woman's pelvic dimensions are unusually small. Common practice used to be to then take X rays to evaluate further the woman's pelvic shape and size. But X rays for this purpose have fallen into disfavor because of their inaccuracy in predicting who will really need a Cesarean. There are a number of important factors in determining the need for a surgical delivery, including some beyond the scope of an X ray. The final size of the fetus and its position, for example, have to be considered; a small baby, well positioned, may be able to fit through where a larger, unusually positioned baby cannot. The strength of the woman's contractions also helps determine whether she will be able to push the baby out vaginally, or will need surgical intervention. A baby who doesn't *look* as if it will get through may actually make it if it molds properly, changing shape as it proceeds down the birth canal.

Obviously, some of those determining factors won't be apparent until the woman is actually in labor. For that reason, most doctors will have such a woman go through what's known as a "trial of labor." Instead of being automatically scheduled for a Cesarean, she will be allowed to go into labor spontaneously, and will be watched closely to see if the baby is descending well and then fitting through the pelvic opening. It may mean a long labor with a prolonged pushing stage, but every attempt is made to achieve vaginal delivery. As one woman describes her experience: "I went through twelve hours of intense labor, with a considerable part of it spent pushing. I tried every position, sitting, squatting, on all fours. I tried everything possible to push the baby out." It turned out that this woman's baby, who weighed almost ten pounds, could not fit through, and a Cesarean was finally performed. But the mother does not regret the effort; she feels that it was worth giving a conventional delivery a try, despite the exhaustion and the pain.

Many times the trials are successful. The baby is not all that big, and the contractions are effective enough to push the baby out of the uterus and then out of the vagina. The point is that accurate prediction is impossible; only after labor has been tried, and has failed, should a Cesarean be done. It is true that bacteria from the vagina frequently travels up to the uterine cavity; thus labor attempts increase the risk of infection if a Cesarean is ultimately performed. But it also has the positive effect of thinning out the lower part of the uterus, where the incision is made, and thus making surgery easier.

Cesareans are sometimes performed for another, more controversial reason—the baby is breech, with its feet or its bottom ready to come out before its head. This is a condition that may be apparent in advance, or may come as a surprise to both doctor and patient. In some cases the doctor discovers it during a routine internal exam toward the end of pregnancy and discusses with the patient what it will mean in terms of the delivery. If there is any doubt about the baby's position, a sonogram will be done to confirm the doctor's findings. But in other cases the breech position isn't discovered until an internal examination during the labor itself. In those instances the baby is probably ready to come out bottom first, and until the cervix is three or four centimeters dilated, the baby's bottom can easily be mistaken for its head. Some women blame their doctors for the lack of advance warning about the breech, but there are often no clues until the labor process is well under way.

When the breech position is discovered, plans are often made for a Cesarean delivery if the woman has not experienced a previous vaginal birth. While it is possible for breech babies to be vaginally delivered by a skilled obstetrician without problems—in fact, at least 95% of the time everything turns out fine—in 3 to 5% of cases a vaginal delivery spells serious trouble for the baby. Since the head is the largest part of the baby, and the last to come out, any significant delay in its emergence could cause brain damage, or localized nerve trauma, or seizures. If it's a really tight squeeze, and the head cannot get through at all, the baby will die. Few if any women informed of those statistics would choose a vaginal delivery, with its small but serious risk to their baby. The risks are the greatest if the baby is in a feet-first position. For a woman who has already given birth vaginally, a vaginal delivery may be attempted with a breech if this second baby is not larger than the first, if its position is not an especially difficult one, and if the doctor is experienced in breech deliveries. Since one baby has already gotten through, there is some confidence that a similar-size baby will also make its way down the birth canal without dangerous delay.

A Second Cesarean?

The most common reason for a woman to have a Cesarean delivery—and the most controversial—is that she has had one before. This is an issue of special relevance to women over 35 because they are the likeliest to have had previous Cesarean births. In most hospitals, until quite recently, one Cesarean delivery automatically meant another. The practice was based on the fear that labor contractions would cause the uterus to rupture along the scar left by the previous Cesarean. But the risk of rupture has declined dramatically as the operative procedure has changed. Instead of performing a "classical" Cesarean, which involves a vertical incision in the upper part of the uterus, doctors now almost invariably make a horizontal incision in the lower segment of the uterus. That type of incision is a safer one, associated with lower maternal and fetal death rates as well as with a lower chance of future rupture. Even if rupture does occur, the critics of "automatic repeats" contend, it usually means just a slight separation of the scar; only when abnormal labor is allowed to progress, without intervention, would a dangerous rupture occur.

There are situations in which repeat Cesareans are mandatory. If the incision was a "classical" one, a vaginal delivery would be too risky to chance. For a woman to know, for certain, what type of uterine incision she had, she should be sure that her medical records are checked; the scar on her abdomen could be misleading. In many instances, the reason for the first Cesarean is present again, and there's no choice but to do another one. For example, if the first Cesarean was for cephalopelvic disproportion, the situation would probably be similar, unless the second baby is considerably smaller than the first.

But very often the original situation does *not* repeat itself. If the first Cesarean was done because of placental separation, multiple birth, a nonprogressing labor, a breech position, or fetal distress—so-called "nonrecurring" reasons—many doctors will put the woman through a trial of labor to see whether a vaginal delivery will be safe. A report by a National Institutes of Health task force supported that practice, advising doctors not to rule out conventional delivery in appropriate cases under appropriate circumstances. The "appropriate circumstances" proviso means that an emergency Cesarean would be possible if anything were to go wrong during labor. To assure that, the labor should take place in a fully equipped medical center with an open blood bank, a full-time anesthesiologist on duty for deliveries, and a full-time operating room (ideally on the same floor as the labor room). A growing number of hospitals with such facilities do allow trials of labor, and their success rate is encouraging. Of the women who undergo such trials, half or more go on to have safe, vaginal births. The chances are best if the cervix has softened and begun to dilate before the labor, and if the baby is in a favorable position, with its head properly descended.

The decision to have a second Cesarean, or to try for a vaginal delivery instead, is not an easy one to make—but it would not be necessary if the *first* Cesarean had not been done. So that is a decision that should not be made automatically, either. While the reason for it may be clear-cut, there are also situations in which a "judgment call" is made, with different doctors making different decisions. A woman should be alert to her doctor's attitude because a Cesarean should never be done casually. It does involve considerably more risks than does a vaginal birth. For the mother, there is a greater chance of infection, of hemorrhage, of a blood clot traveling to the lung. There are also the risks that go along with a major anesthetic being used, and the pain and discomfort that follow abdominal surgery.

Critics charge that some Cesareans are performed unnecessarily. They say that doctors are no longer being trained to perform difficult deliveries, and so they sometimes turn too readily to a surgical solution. One real impetus to a high Cesarean rate is the fear of malpractice suits. Many doctors are afraid that a decision *not* to do a Cesarean in a borderline situation could come back to haunt them both legally and financially if the vaginal delivery doesn't go well. The use of fetal monitors has also been pointed to as causing a rush to Cesareans; critics contend that doctors sometimes misinterpret changes in the fetal heartbeat pattern, and therefore perform unjustified surgical deliveries. As we've discussed earlier in the book, that may have been true when fetal monitors were first being used, but increasing experience with them, and growing medical understanding of fetal heartbeat patterns, have lessened that risk.

The major role you can play in avoiding an unnecessary Cesarean is to ask physicians the right questions before you select one, or to question your doctor carefully during your early visits. If the doctor seems to consider a woman over 35 a high-risk patient just for being over 35, that may spell a Cesarean in your future. If the Cesarean rate that he or she quotes seems high to you, it may mean that the practice has a lot of high-risk patients, or that some Cesareans are being done for no good reason. In discussing the issue together you may get an idea of the reason behind the high number and a grasp of just what this physician's approach to Cesareans is. Another question to ask your doctor is whether he or she gets a second opinion before performing a Cesarean delivery. This is a practice that is recommended by the American College of Obstetricians and Gynecologists and is the policy in a growing number of medical centers. It is an important safeguard against unnecessary Cesareans. (In extreme emergency situations, such as hemorrhage or severe fetal distress, a Cesarean can be legitimately performed without another doctor's concurrence.) If you raise and discuss the issue of Cesareans early in your doctor-patient relationship, the trust that develops between you will be beneficial should a difficult decision be necessary later in your pregnancy.

The Time to Prepare

A Cesarean is not something that any pregnant woman looks forward to, but it is something that every pregnant woman should be ready for. Women over 35, in particular, should not assume that their delivery will be vaginal, because the chances are one in four that it won't be. Even the most perfect pregnancy can come to its conclusion on an operating table. The better the pregnancy has been going, the worse the shock of the Cesarean can be. "Mine was a model pregnancy, and I expected a model birth," recalled a woman three months after her Cesarean delivery. "I thought it would be easy, that my baby would just fall out. Both my mother and grandmother had easy, short labors, so why not me? When I found out the baby was breech and I would need a Cesarean, it was just so unexpected. I was shocked and disappointed. Everything that I had learned at Lamaze, everything that I had practiced, was for nothing now. I was sorry that I had bothered."

It can be frustrating to have attended classes in preparation for a birth experience that will never be, but those classes can be useful even for women who will have, whether they know it or not, a Cesarean delivery. Many women tend to tune out any information pertaining to a Cesarean, to look elsewhere if a film depicting a Cesarean is shown in class, to skip over any written material that describes this other method of childbirth. They think, and hope, that it just can't happen to them. But it can, and they should be prepared for it by learning the facts. The facts are available in preparation classes and in books; to listen and to learn what a Cesarean entails is as important as is the practice and preparation for a vaginal delivery, especially for women in the over-35, Cesarean-prone age group.

If you know ahead of time that you will definitely be having a Cesarean childbirth, you'll have more intensive preparation to do. You may want to read books that focus exclusively on Cesarean births, as well as talk to other women who have gone through a Cesarean experience. You'll want to ask your obstetrician to acquaint you with the particular procedures in the hospital where you'll be delivering. Once a Cesarean is scheduled, there are a number of issues you should bring up with your doctor: What should you do if you experience the beginning signs of labor before the scheduled surgery? What type of anesthesia will you be receiving? What type of incision will be done? Will your husband be allowed to remain with you throughout the surgery? Will you be able to nurse the baby on the operating table? Will you be able to spend time together as a family after the surgery? Again, as with a vaginal delivery, your views may have an influence on some of the aspects of the procedure—for example, your preference for an epidural or spinal anesthetic that will allow you to remain awake, or for a general anesthetic that will put you completely out; your desire to nurse the baby immediately; your desire for a family time after the baby's birth. With your input, the Cesarean delivery of your baby can turn into a fulfilling and satisfying birth experience, a shared experience for all your family.

But before you focus on the positive, you'll have some negatives to get through. Some of them will come from other people, people who haven't been through it themselves, and are well-meaning but full of misinformation. Sandy, a woman in her thirties who was scheduled for a Cesarean due to the breech position of her baby, was frightened about facing the surgery. The thoughtless comments of others only served to intensify her fear: "There was a sort of sadness in the people around me. When I told them about the Cesarean, they expressed pity for me. 'Oh, that's terrible.' That kind of reaction was just not merited. And it bred my own negative feelings." The hospital was insensitive to her needs, as well. The hospital tour taken by her preparation class focused only on vaginal births. Cesareans were not addressed, and the facilities for them not shown. When Sandy asked what the operating room would be like, the tour guide replied, "Did you see *Coma* and *M*A*S*H*? The rooms look just like that." That response did not sit well with Sandy. "I was very upset. I hadn't associated that type of environment with giving birth. I thought it was horrible." Thoughtless comments can be devastating, if you let them get to you. It's important to remember that things will *not* be as bad as some people portray them. In fact, Sandy considered the operating room where her baby was later born to be just fine. "There was nothing scary about it. It even had a window in it of glazed glass. It was not intimidating at all." Comments needn't be intimidating, either, if you let them pass over you, and heed only those that are sensible and well informed.

It is possible to dismiss the irrational, insensitive opinions of others—but not so easy to dismiss your own feelings of shock and disappointment. Those are common reactions to an impending Cesarean, shock that such a "perfect" pregnancy should come to this unwelcome end, disappointment that all the preparation for a vaginal delivery was apparently for naught. There is commonly a feeling of failure, that your body has let you down, that if you had done something differently perhaps this wouldn't be happening to you. Many women go through a grieving period from the time they learn that a Cesarean is necessary. They are grieving for the experience that they won't be having; they are grieving for their wasted energies and their dashed hopes. "I felt a real loss when I learned the birth would be Cesarean," said one mother, who had worked long and hard in preparation for a vaginal delivery. "I had learned Lamaze. I had taken it seriously. I practiced it when I could have been doing something else. I did everything I was supposed to do for my baby. When I found out I wouldn't be having a natural birth I felt a loss. I was going to miss out on something I had been planning on and counting on for a long time."

For many women, particularly experienced career women who are used to having some control over their lives, the news of a Cesarean can signal the loss of that control. "Everything in my life was very well organized," relates a 36-year-old first-time mother. "I delayed childbearing until I felt that everything was under control. I was happily married. I had a good, regular kind of job after years of working crazy shifts. Now I was working normal hours, and my life was in order. I decided that it was finally time to have a child. So I became pregnant—and that was the beginning of the end of the control. If the baby was kicking, I got no sleep. If it was leaning on my bladder, I spent most of my time in the bathroom. I tried to get part of the control back by preparing myself for the labor. I went to all the classes, I did the breathing, I did the exercises. But then I learned I'd be having a Cesarean, and I lost the control all over again. I knew that I wouldn't be doing the breathing. I knew that I wouldn't be controlling the birth of my child. It was so sudden and unexpected. I had been used to managing my life. Now my life was managing me."

But to look at it more positively, the lost sense of control may be replaced by an added sense of certainty. The birth of your child will likely be a scheduled one. The odds are that it will not catch you unprepared, nor leave you with your suitcase packed but nowhere to go. The date you circle on your calendar will most probably be the date your baby will be born. Also, while you may have less control over the birth process, you will have a more accurate idea of exactly what the process will entail. Vaginal births are full of unknowns while Cesarean births generally go exactly according to plan. You'll know, ahead of time, the order of events, approximately how long the delivery will take, just when you'll be holding your new baby in your arms.

You'll also know that in some very important ways a Cesarean birth can be similar to a more natural experience. Two issues are paramount in the minds of many women facing Cesarean deliveries: Will I be awake when my baby is born? Will my husband be with me during the delivery prccess? For more and more women, the answers to both those questions are "yes." For Cesarean deliveries the favored form of anesthesia among most women is now regional (an epidural or spinal), which leaves the woman pain-free but alert to her surroundings and to the events of the birth. And part of her surroundings will likely be her husband, as increasing numbers of hospitals are allowing fathers into operating rooms as well as into delivery rooms. Such affirmative answers make the anticipation of a Cesarean less of a blow, less of a loss. Says one woman who recently went through the Cesarean experience, "When it was clear that I wouldn't miss out on being awake, and holding the baby, and having my husband present, I was less disappointed about missing out on one of life's experiences. I knew that the essence of what I wanted would be there."

Any disappointment in facing a Cesarean will be tempered in the woman who concentrates more on the fate of her baby than on the experience of giving birth. Despite the innovations, a Cesarean childbirth does fall short of a vaginal birth, and the recovery period is more difficult. But the major goal of the surgery is not to fulfill the mother's expectations; rather, it is to ensure the baby's healthy survival. Undergoing a Cesarean when it's medically indicated is the very best thing you can be doing for your baby, a gift of life and good health from mother to child.

The Scheduled Cesarean

Once the decision has been made to have a Cesarean, the date for the procedure will be set. Although it may tentatively be scheduled for a few days before a woman's due date, the appointment may be changed according to the progress of the pregnancy. Sometimes scientific measures are employed, such as a sonogram, to judge the size and maturity of the fetus and the maturity of the placenta, or an amniocentesis is done to determine whether the baby's lungs are mature. The aim is to schedule the surgery *before* labor starts spontaneously but *after* the baby is ready to cope with the outside world. In most cases, that's just what happens. The mother goes into the hospital by appointment and comes out with a fully mature baby.

The general procedure for a scheduled Cesarean is for the woman to check into the hospital the night before or the morning of the surgery. She'll be told not to drink or eat anything after midnight— a standard, presurgical prohibition intended to prevent problems under anesthesia. One of the first things she'll face on the day of the surgery will be the starting of an intravenous line to administer fluid. The top of her pubic hair will probably be shaved off and a catheter may be inserted to drain her bladder. An epidural anesthetic may be started a half hour or longer before the scheduled surgery. If a spinal or general anesthetic is being used, it would be given closer to the time that surgery is scheduled. The abdomen will be rubbed with an antiseptic solution prior to the start of the surgery. Even if a woman is awake with an epidural or spinal anesthetic, she may be given an oxygen mask to wear until the baby is born. In most hospitals a drape or a screen is then put in place to block the mother's view of the surgery; some doctors maintain that such a barrier also provides a sterile field, but others are willing to dispense with it at the mother's request. At this point in the proceedings the father may be brought in to share in the actual birth experience (if he's allowed in, if he wants to be there, and if his wife is conscious). He generally sits right beside his wife so that he can be a real emotional support for her. His role is to be with her, *not* to witness the actual surgery, and so he is also positioned behind the screen. In some hospitals, though, he is not allowed even that close, and may be relegated to a glass booth some distance from his wife. She may barely feel his presence, although it is some improvement over his total banishment from the birthing.

Kathryn remembers well the first Cesarean she performed with a father present. She had been performing the surgery for years at that time, but her experience didn't prevent her from feeling anxious that this very interested observer was in the room. He was much older than she was, and was seeing his wife through her second Cesarean. Kathryn felt quite insecure about his watching over her shoulder. She was careful to do a very good job, meticulously tying every knot. But when she spoke with him after the procedure, he told her he had paid no attention to her surgical technique. He had been concentrating on being with his wife and new baby as an active participant in the birth event. After that experience, Kathryn never again felt anxious with a father in the operating room. On the contrary, she felt that he was an exciting addition to the delivery experience.

The Cesarean surgery itself is comprised of first an incision in the various layers of the abdominal wall, then an incision in the uterine wall, followed by the delivery of the baby and the placenta. The baby is usually delivered within ten minutes of the initial incision, and sometimes even sooner than that. While there is typically another thirty or thirty-five minutes of the surgery to go, many couples barely notice it because now they have their baby. The Cesarean fades into the background as they focus on the life they created. Cesarean babies are as a whole a beautiful bunch, unbruised and unmolded by a long, torturous labor. Disappointment at the manner of birth can turn into delight at its result with just a single glance. "I was so excited when I saw her, I just cried," recalls the mother of a newborn Cesarean baby. "She was just gorgeous. She was big and had a full head of hair." Another mother, looking back three months to the birth of her daughter, remembers her reaction to her baby more vividly than she does the Cesarean itself. "It was a big surprise to me. I didn't expect to think of my baby as so beautiful and so wonderful. She's just a little cherub. In my memory of the whole thing, the Cesarean really has very little moment. So I went through a little pain. When I look at my daughter I realize that the way of giving birth is really not so important."

Looking at the baby after it's born is not enough for most couples. They want to hold it, and in many hospitals both father and mother are allowed to do so, though the mother may find it a bit awkward. Some mothers even want to nurse the baby while still on the operating table, and there is no medical or logical reason why that shouldn't be possible, though it too can be somewhat awkward. While all this looking, and holding, and nursing is going on, the surgical team is finishing up their work, tying up blood vessels, putting things back in place, closing up the incisions. The outer incision is closed either with stitches that will have to be removed, with dissolving stitches, or with staples. One woman, now the mother of a two-month-old girl, remembers chatting with the doctor throughout this part of the operation and asking him exactly what he was doing as he was sewing. When he started explaining the surgical procedure in graphic detail, she decided that she really didn't want to hear about it, after all. She much preferred hearing the nurses tell her just how beautiful her baby was. The Cesarean may not have been exactly the birth experience she had hoped for, but her daughter was just the baby she wanted.

Cesarean by Surprise

Knowing just when and how the Cesarean will be performed is very reassuring to some women, as they can order their lives around the impending procedure. But some women find the foreknowledge to be downright dull, especially women who know the sex of the baby (through an amniocentesis) as well as the date it will be born. Where's the drama? Where's the excitement? What is left of nature's greatest mystery? Sometimes nature does add a twist to such a pedestrian plot, when the birth process begins before it is "supposed" to; the rush to the hospital may then be even more dramatic than it is for a vaginal birth. It is a rush to get the baby out as planned—by Cesarean—rather than by the vaginal route that has been deemed to be too risky for this particular baby.

If you are scheduled for a Cesarean, you should be aware of the early signs of labor—the contractions, the premature rupture of the membranes, the bloody discharge—and report their onset at once to your physician. You may well find that the Lamaze exercises you had practiced, and then dismissed as a waste of time, do come in handy because you may actually be in labor for several hours (first at home and then at the hospital) before the Cesarean is performed. It will likely be only mild labor, but mild is a relative term, and you may be happy for any help available to you.

If this is your second or subsequent baby, there will be more of a sense of urgency in getting the Cesarean underway, especially if your previous labors were short. If the birth seems imminent you may be whisked into the operating room and given a general anesthetic so the surgery can begin quickly. A general anesthetic may be used in this instance because it is faster acting than an epidural. The initial part of the surgery is speeded up, and the baby is often removed within three or four minutes so that it will not be adversely affected by the anesthetic drug. (In a real emergency, the baby can be removed within a minute.) The surprise aspect of a "too soon" Cesarean can come as a welcome bit of drama in an otherwise predictable proceeding, but the surprise of a general anesthetic is rarely as warmly received. It means the end of virtually all similarities to a vaginal delivery, including (in most hospitals) the presence of the husband, and may prove the ultimate disappointment.

Many Cesarean births begin as normal vaginal deliveries, but something happens along the route that makes the Cesarean the method of choice. It may be a case of unsuspected cephalopelvic disproportion, or of fetal distress resulting from a twisted or knotted umbilical cord (with the baby beyond the reach of forceps). Or, as noted earlier, a baby thought to be head down may be discovered to be breech during the course of the labor. And so a woman totally unprepared for the Cesarean experience becomes a Cesarean mother, perhaps even under the emergency conditions of a general anesthetic. The shock of it can be shattering, the disappointment devastating. She may already have put in hours and hours of excruciatingly painful labor. This is not at all what she had in mind, and she may translate her own feelings of failure into anger at those around her. In fact, some doctors apologize when they announce the need for a Cesarean, perhaps to ward off such a hostile, angry reaction. But there are women who react much differently. Belle was one of them: "I was in labor so long, and it was very, very difficult. Despite all my efforts at pushing, the baby was just too large to come out. When I found out I'd be having a Cesarean I had mixed feelings about it. In one way I was relieved. Anything was better than the pain I was feeling. The first thing I said was 'Get the man with the drugs.' I didn't think clearly in terms of goals or the next step. All I thought of was being out of the pain." The differing reactions are based largely on a woman's perceived contribution to the event. If she feels that the Cesarean was biologically determined, and outside of her control, she may have a more accepting attitude. But if she considers herself in any way responsible for it—by taking an anesthetic drug, for example, or by not pushing hard enough—then the emotional trauma of the event may last long beyond the baby's birth.

The Road to Recovery

Belle's relief at the cessation of pain was actually a bit premature. While the actual period of the surgery was a pain-free interlude, the pain returned in different form not long after, combined with an array of discomforts typical of the post-Cesarean period. Many women who are fully prepared for the surgery itself are totally unprepared for what comes after.

The immediate aftermath of a Cesarean involves a stay in the recovery room, often *without* husband and baby. That can be a very difficult time for a woman still high on the thrill of the birth, a time of separation from her newly formed family. "It was very lonely in there," remembers one new mother. "I felt completely deserted. I was just lying there, not knowing what was happening. I begged the nurses to let me go. Finally, after two hours, they wheeled me to my room. When I got there I was greeted by the sight of my husband sitting on a chair, reading a newspaper, with the baby on his lap. One look at them helped to compensate for the wait." It may be worth discussing this recovery period with your doctor, finding out if a significant time of separation really is necessary. Perhaps your physician will be willing to modify the standard procedure for you—or will be able to convince you of the rationale behind the way things are usually done. If you do find yourself alone in recovery, lonely for your family, try to focus on the sight and touch of your newborn baby, and all the joy your baby will soon be bringing you. You won't be lonely for long!

Once you're out of the recovery room, you'll be able to spend more time with your baby, but that doesn't mean that your recovery is over. You're in for a recovery period that is longer and harder than one from a vaginal birth. In one way, that is allowed for; your scheduled stay in the hospital will be five to seven days, compared to two to four days after a conventional delivery. But in other ways, the expectations of hospital staff, friends, and family may not be in line with what you're really going through. You may be made to feel that you're not progressing fast enough, that you're not performing well enough, that your inadequacy in needing a Cesarean is matched by your inadequacy in getting over it. Such feelings may be further fueled by the sight of the energetic endeavors of your non-Cesarean roommates. Three days after Barbara's Cesarean, she was still lying in bed most of the time, back up, feet raised, unable to do anything without the utmost concentration. Only seven hours before, her roommate Claire gave birth vaginally, and Barbara was all too aware of the differences between them. "Here she was showering, eating breakfast, hopping around.

I told her I couldn't believe it, that she's just incredible. The speed of her recovery was marvelous, but it just pointed up the slowness of mine."

There is no reason for a woman to blame herself for a "too slow" recovery; it is in the nature of the surgery and its medical aftermath. There will be a number of physical reminders that what did transpire was indeed major surgery. After the Cesarean, a woman is hooked up for several days to an IV, which contains either a dextrose and water or salt water solution, plus oxytocin to contract the uterus. She'll also be given pain-relieving medication for two or three days, most often Demerol or morphine, and then milder-acting pills, such as codeine, aspirin, or acetaminophen. The early pain she feels will be from the incision itself; later it will be gas pains that cause her the most distress. In fact, the very word "gas" may begin to be a pain in itself. It's a word a woman begins to hear very often on the second or third day after surgery as doctors and nurses alike ask her whether she's passed any. "When you're in bed, your progress is measured by whether you passed gas or not," recalls Cathy all too vividly, though three months have gone by since she was put to the test. "All you can eat until you pass gas is bouillon, jello, and ginger ale, no real solids. It's the key to your freedom. You're not a human being until you pass gas." This apparent obsession may seem cruel to hungry patients, but it's an important clue to their medical progress. After the surgery their intestines are temporarily paralyzed. If they eat too soon they may vomit, and the process of recovery will be slowed down. The passing of gas is an indication that the muscular movement of the digestive system is working properly—and that eating can be both satisfying *and* safe. One woman said that she was tempted to lie in this area "to get the nurses off my back," but that would only have produced more problems for her, retarding her recovery instead of producing the normalcy she wanted.

Another reality of the post-Cesarean period is the bladder catheter and its aftereffects. It may be left in for up to twenty-four hours after the surgery, a period some women are not too happy about, but others would like to see extended. "The catheter was very convenient," says one, "because I didn't have to get up to go to the bathroom. And getting up was not easy. I was sorry when they took it out." Many women feel an area of vaginal irritation when the catheter is removed, and most have some trouble urinating (a frequent problem after a vaginal delivery as well). Because these catheters can cause bladder infections, urine cultures are commonly done after the catheter is removed.

Whether it's to go to the bathroom, or simply to sit up in bed, moving around is not easy for the first few days after a Cesarean. It's painful, and difficult, and just plain exhausting. Even once a woman is standing, she may not be able to stand up straight, and she may find herself walking in the "Cesarean shuffle," a funny name for a very unfunny situation. Too tired, or embarrassed, to do it, she may remain, unmoving, in bed. But she is not helping herself get better. It's important to move around, once the doctor permits it, as a way to get the gas moving quicker and to clear out the lungs. It's something a woman has to force herself to do, but she'll be a step closer to recovery for it. Periodic deep breathing is another aspect of recovery that may hurt to even *think* of doing, but will help prevent the pulmonary complications that can occur after abdominal surgery and anesthesia.

After a Cesarean, the awkwardness and the difficulty in moving about can be particularly frustrating because there is someone else beside yourself to think about—your baby. You may find it hard to care for your new baby, or to lift it. The women who manage best are the ones who are not afraid to ask for help from their visitors as well as from the hospital staff. Someone can help you to sit up, can hand you the baby, can provide a secure presence as you hold your baby, lovingly and as steadily as you can. An electric bed, which you can operate by pushing a button, will also help you to get into position for maneuvering yourself and your baby, and you should ask your doctor ahead of time if one can be made available for you. Your feeling of awkwardness will probably last only about two days, but there's no need to miss out on the first two days of your baby's life.

Nor is there a need to miss out on the beginning of the breast-feeding experience. Although the milk comes in about a day later after a Cesarean delivery than after a vaginal one, there are both medical and psychological advantages to getting an early start on the nursing relationship. Some women have no particular problem with it, nursing on the operating table and regularly after that. Others find it difficult because of the pain of the incision, and have to experiment to find a comfortable position; many women who have undergone Cesareans find it easiest to nurse sitting up in a chair. Again, being willing to ask for help is a big bonus—help in being handed the baby, help in switching the baby from one side to the other. An electric bed will also help you to get into a comfortable position for breast-feeding. The help you will need is only temporary; the benefits to be gained are long-lasting.

The recovery period from a Cesarean is difficult, but the worst of its physical aspects are over in two or three days. Each day after that will bring with it a remarkable improvement, and before you know it you'll feel little the worse for the surgery. About five days after the delivery, your stitches or staples will be removed—a sign that you are almost ready to leave the hospital. By then you probably won't be envying your non-Cesarean roommates so much. In fact, you may feel sympathy for their episiotomy pain and their hemorrhoidal discomforts. Most of *your* pain was of a higher order—and most of it is over. Within a month to six weeks of your surgery, you will feel physically yourself again, aside from the rigors of taking care of your baby.

The emotional pain of a Cesarean can last longer, however, sometimes lingering even past the baby's first birthday. The feelings of disappointment, and loss, and grief, can be the most tenacious in women whose Cesarean was a surprise, and who didn't have the chance to work through those emotions before the birth. Not until they have gotten past the physical demands of recovery can they begin to come to terms with the psychological aspects. One of the most difficult feelings to shake is that of guilt—if only I had been braver my baby would have been spared the Cesarean.

The best way to deal with the self-blame is to find out the facts about your case. Ask your doctor just why the Cesarean was necessary. Go over what you think your part may have been in it, for example, that you hadn't been a diligent enough Lamaze student, or that your pushing was more feeble than forceful. Most likely you'll find out that you bear no responsibility whatever for the Cesarean. An emotion that sometimes grows with the passing weeks is anger, anger that you were deprived of a vaginal birth, anger that you may direct at the medical personnel involved in the Cesarean decision. You may have very legitimate questions about how that decision was made, and even about how your medical care may have somehow contributed to the need for a Cesarean. This is no time to be shy about your doubts or suspicions. Do ask the relevant questions of the involved personnel, and perhaps read the books on Cesarean deliveries you hadn't read before, so that you can intelligently assess their answers. The chances are that you'll find that your course of treatment was correct and that the Cesarean was the best or only delivery option. Then you'll be able to deal with your anger on a more realistic basis, and eventually let it go. If you find out otherwise, you can express your anger directly, at the responsible parties, and resolve to choose a different medical team for your future gynecological and obstetrical needs.

Because of the emotional aftermath so common to Cesarean births, numerous parents' support groups have been formed. Here parents can discuss their common concerns and help each other deal with their feelings. These groups are invaluable resources for parents who may feel alone in their emotions, stigmatized by a form of birth they didn't expect, didn't want, and still can't get over. Your obstetrician or childbirth education instructor can direct you to a support group or to another resource, "Cesarean Talk Lines," which are also being developed to meet the emotional needs of Cesarean patients.

Many of these groups focus on the future as well as on the past, providing information on the option of attempting a vaginal delivery after a Cesarean. For women who are planning to have another child, and who can realistically think in terms of a trial of labor, that hope can help to dull their present pain. But even for women with no new baby in sight, or with a definite Cesarean in their reproductive future, there is an overriding reason for optimism. That optimism involves the baby they already have. Research has revealed no long-term negative effects on child development as the outcome of a Cesarean birth. The challenge is for the parents to stop dwelling on the disappointing aspects of the birth, to stop thinking of how it *might* have been, and to focus their attention on this most beautiful of babies.

13

Coming Home:
Your New Baby, Your New Life

The day you give birth is the day you become a mother, but you may feel your new role most keenly on the day you take your baby home. As you dress your baby, excitedly, in the outfit you chose so carefully for this special occasion, and as you dress yourself, with some distaste, in the only clothes that are likely to fit you—your maternity clothes—you are apt to feel a wave of mixed emotions. On one hand, there is the thrill of taking charge of this bundle of new life, of removing it from the nurses' care into your own care, of crossing the threshold of your home with your baby in your arms. Now you'll be able to do things *your* way, without the intervention of the hospital staff in the care of your baby, without the routine of the nurses to rule the rhythms of your life. But even as you're savoring your "release" from institutional life, you may also experience another emotion—the fear of handling motherhood outside the reassuring safety of the hospital environment. The nurses may have been intrusive, but at least they knew what they were doing. Many new mothers are not so sure about their own abilities. They wonder just how they'll be able to nurture the tiny life now in their charge. They feel overwhelmed by their new responsibility, fearful that they'll fail. And so they may view their discharge from the hospital not so much as a release from confinement as a sentence to a job for which they are eminently unqualified.

Leaving the hospital is a mother's moment of truth, and whether you face it with eagerness or with anxiety will depend largely on your previous experience in the role of caretaker and on your preparations for your future role. Women who have already tended to babies, whether younger siblings, or neighbors' children, or nieces or nephews, generally approach the future with confidence—much more so than women who have never changed a diaper or even held a baby before. There is little opportunity in this society to learn about parenting except from direct experience, and that experience eludes many women until they're sent home from the hospital with diapers, formula, and their very own baby. One way to make up for the lack is to take a course in baby care *before* the baby is on the scene, sometime in the latter half of your pregnancy. Your doctor or childbirth educator can probably direct you to such a course, or your local Red Cross chapter may offer one. It can be hard to see beyond the pregnancy and the birth experience to the baby's requirements for care, but some preparation will help in your transition from expectant parenthood to motherhood, and will make coming home a more joyful experience.

Finding Help During the First Weeks at Home

One way to alleviate the transition to new motherhood is to arrange for help during the first weeks at home. Even if you feel quite capable of cooking and cleaning and, with your coursework behind you, even of mothering, now is not the time to exert yourself in a show of superwomanly stamina. When your baby cries for you, you may find yourself crying for help. It's best to arrange for help before the birth, when you still have the time and energy to consider intelligently what your needs will be.

One alternative available to some women is to ask a relative to stay with them for the first week or two after the birth. Your mother may offer to move in to help you out in this most trying of times. Since she is the one with the "experience" in baby care, she may take it upon herself to do most of the actual mothering, as well as to lay down the rules and regulations of proper baby care. But you and your mother can run into trouble that way, and so can your baby if arguments ensue over how best to cope with its needs. You've probably developed certain ideas through reading, or talking with friends, about the way you would like to do things in these early weeks—ideas that may clash with your mother's way of doing things. As an over-35 woman, long independent of your parents, you may bridle at your mother's attempts at control. Although you may certainly benefit from suggestions or guidance from your mother, it is you who should flex your "mothering" muscles and assume the major care of the baby, as well as the decision-making. Only by giving the baby a bath, changing its diaper, comforting it in its distress, will you gain the confidence to be the mother you know you can be. And your mother can still play an important role, doing errands for you, preparing meals, being available as a source of knowledge and experience.

When mother and daughter each play the appropriate role, they can discover a new side to their relationship, and enjoy each other in an unexpected way. "My mother and I are always on each other's nerves, but this time was much different," relates Andrea, whose mother had spent the first two postpartum weeks with her daughter's new family. "Although I was the baby's main caretaker, she was a great help. That extra pair of hands made a difference. She cooked, she helped clean, she gave the baby a relief bottle. This was the only time in my life I was together with her for so long without having a single fight. She was just terrific. As much as anything, I enjoyed her company."

But some women are certain that they *won't* enjoy their mother's company, or their mother or another close relative isn't available, or they feel guilty asking for a lot of help and would rather pay for it. And so they think in terms of professional assistance. Here, again, the same principle applies: better to care for the baby yourself, to get to really know your newborn from the start of its life, and to hire someone to do the *other* work around the house. That someone—whom you may be able to find through an agency specializing in household help—can spell you with the baby at times, but will mainly take care of the chores that you won't have the time or the energy to do. Depending on your financial state and on your inclination, this can be someone who comes in for either a few mornings or afternoons a week or who spends all day with you. Ideally, it is someone you interview and hire before your baby's birth so you can approach with equanimity your first weeks as a mother.

For some new mothers, no one less than a baby nurse will do.

They are terrified at the thought of taking care of a new infant, too insecure to take on the job alone when the child is at its most vulnerable. They need to know that the baby is in good hands—someone else's hands. And so they hire a baby nurse for a week or more, perhaps for as long as they can afford one, putting off the day when the baby's care becomes their responsibility. For women who are very unsure about their caretaking capabilities, this may be the best way to alleviate anxiety, if they go about it the right way. Other women, more secure in their mothering abilities, may choose a baby nurse because they have older children to care for, or other responsibilities, and want to be able to fit in some time to rest and relax. If you decide this is the best choice for you, you might ask your obstetrician or pediatrician for a recommendation, or hire someone through an agency specializing in baby nurses. If possible, interview baby nurses ahead of time to find one whose personality and baby care philosophy complement your own. If you intend to breast-feed, determine whether the nurse will support you in your feeding efforts. Her enthusiasm or lack of it in this regard will indicate how she will act on the job—whether she will give you the encouragement you need as you initiate nursing, or will seem overly eager to stick a bottle in your baby's mouth, asserting her authority at the expense of your efforts.

One thing you should make clear, before hiring someone, is that part of her job will be to teach you how to take care of the baby. You should consider the nurse's stay as an apprenticeship period for you, as a time for learning the ropes; otherwise, you'll be left at the end of her stay as terrified as you were at the beginning, scared of being left alone with your own child. If the nurse does not seem cooperative in your learning efforts, or your feeding efforts, or is very disappointing in other ways, you should consider either hiring another nurse or hiring a housekeeper instead. If you let things continue as they are, you'll only feel more stressed by your current nurse's presence, and she won't be doing you or your baby any good.

Arranging for help is particularly important for a mother who is single. As the only parent at home, she can be easily overwhelmed by the demands of new parenthood, and needs someone who can help share the burden. It can be a friend or relative who can help out on a regular basis or, if she can afford it, a competent housekeeper. A reliable support system is especially important to her because of her situation: She'll need someone to take care of the baby if she's sick, and she'll need someone to babysit when she leaves to go to work, as most single mothers do. It's not only the early weeks after the birth she'll have to consider in hiring household and child care help; she'll also have to set up a backup support system to operate on a continuing basis.

The Physical Transition

If you think that it sounds like too much trouble to enlist help—that you would just as soon give it a go yourself—think again. The main consideration is that you won't really *be* yourself for the first few weeks after your baby is born. Shedding your baby and some weight does not mean that you'll get your prepregnancy body back so soon, with all your old stamina and energy. In fact, some women find the postpartum period even more physically uncomfortable than the pregnancy. "I really felt well when I was pregnant," recalls one woman, two months after the birth of her first child and her own fortieth birthday. "Pregnancy was such a satisfying, content, wonderful experience. But after the birth my body felt draggy. I ached in all of my joints and muscles. I felt terribly out of shape and moved awkwardly, much more so than toward the end of the pregnancy. It was a whole new physiological adjustment. It wasn't easy, and there was no feeling of contentment."

During the early weeks at home with your baby, you'll still be experiencing some of the physical discomforts that began after the birth. Although your episiotomy stitches will have dissolved within two weeks of delivery, there'll still be some pulling and healing for another two or three weeks after that. Your vaginal discharge will change from bloody red to the creamier, more brownish "lochia," also within about two weeks of the delivery. Your uterus continues to shrink for several weeks, going down in size from about one and one-half pounds following the birth to its normal weight of two ounces, though the afterpains become less painful with the passage of time. If you developed hemorrhoids during late pregnancy, you may find that they continue to be a nuisance for a couple of months after the birth. But those changes (which are discussed more fully in chapter 12), are just part of the post-pregnancy transition—a transition made far more rapidly than the physical transition into the pregnancy state. Another common change is edema, or swelling of the legs. It can happen even in women who experienced no edema during pregnancy, and is a result of the sudden and drastic change in the body's fluid balance after the birth of the baby. Edema can come as an unwelcome surprise to a woman who hasn't had it before, but it is nothing to be alarmed about, and generally goes away within two weeks of delivery.

Breast changes can also persist past the day of homecoming, as the breasts remain hard, and full, and uncomfortable. For non-nursing mothers, some relief can be attained through breast binders (see page 189). For nursing mothers, the discomfort will probably continue for the first weeks at home, but will gradually diminish as the nursing becomes well established. The best course is to stick with it, to accept the difficulties as temporary, to feel confident that things will get easier and even quite enjoyable. If you experience any difficulty, particularly if you develop a fever, or an area of redness in the breast, or if the breast feels hot and is tender to the touch, you should let your doctor know about it. You may have developed a breast infection, which doesn't mean that you need to stop nursing, but does require medical attention.

Another common problem for nursing mothers is sore or cracked nipples. A remedy Kathryn has recommended to many of her patients involves squeezing a small amount of A and D ointment onto a circle of wax paper; the circle should be big enough to cover the whole nipple area. Put the circle into your tightest bra, and wear it in between nursing sessions. When it's time to nurse, peel off the paper but leave the ointment on. After nursing, begin the "wax paper" treatment again. The soreness and cracks are generally gone within twenty-four hours. Most breast-feeding problems—cracked nipples, sluggish milk flow, sucking difficulties—occur within the first few weeks. It's a matter of mother and baby getting used to breast-feeding and adjusting to each other's rhythms. But don't get discouraged. Things generally do get easier. And don't rush to supplement with bottles if you plan to nurse full-time for a number of months. Have patience and confidence in the breast-feeding process, and you'll soon find it a lot of fun.

One change most pregnant women anticipate with eagerness is a drastic loss in weight and a return to their prepregnancy profiles. There will, certainly, be some weight loss after the birth, usually twelve to fifteen pounds within just a couple of days, and up to another ten pounds within the next week. But some women find that five pounds or so just seem to stick with them, weight that keeps them from fitting comfortably into their old clothes. And most of the extra weight seems, unhappily, to cling to their mid-section. Not only may they still look pregnant for a while, they may have to resort to their already well-worn maternity wardrobe. The reason is not only that they weigh more than usual, but that their abdominal muscles have loosened and their skin stretched out to accommodate the extra bulk of the pregnancy. The results can be distressing. One woman, a week after delivery, took her first walk out of the house to pick up some baby supplies. An onlooker made a statement that she had heard many times during the pregnancy: "It's going to be a boy!" She turned to him and said, "It *was* a boy." She didn't wait around to see the astonished look on his face—but she did wait quite a while before she ventured outside again. Her experience may have been unusual but her feelings are not unique. Research has found that dissatisfaction with one's appearance is often more intense during the postpartum period than during the pregnancy itself.

A realistic remedy to the situation involves a combination of patience, good diet, and light exercise. If weight gain during pregnancy was not excessive, virtually all of it usually comes off within the first few weeks after the birth. It's best to eat a well-balanced diet during that period in order to keep up your health and your energy; if you're nursing, you'll need to consume a higher-than-normal quantity of protein, calories, and liquids to support your milk production as well as to meet your own nutritional needs. For women who have gained more than thirty pounds during the pregnancy, some of that weight may remain, and prove hard to shed. But this is not the time to go on a crash reduction diet, with all the physical and psychological stresses you'll be undergoing. Rather, it's the perfect time for a sensible weight-reduction plan, ideally under your physician's supervision.

A mild exercise program, focusing on strengthening the abdominal muscles, can also help to eliminate the pregnancy look that is not exactly ego-enhancing to the new mother. Some good exercises for this period are leg lifts and sit-ups. You may find that you can only do partial sit-ups for the first few weeks—perhaps only getting your head and shoulders off the floor—but that's enough to accomplish the tightening you're aiming for. As time passes, you'll gradually find yourself approaching a full sit-up. This exercise regimen should be started soon after the birth, but it should not become so vigorous as to produce excessive vaginal bleeding. If bleeding does increase during or subsequent to the exercise session, that's a signal to slow down, that more healing must take place before strenuous exercise is in order.

The After-Baby Blues

All the physical changes that accompany and follow birth seem to affect a woman's psyche as well as her body. Most women experience what's been termed "postpartum blues," beginning anywhere from the third to the seventh day after delivery. Scientists conjecture that this state of sadness, weepiness, and irritability is the result of changing levels of the hormones estrogen and progesterone, as well as other chemical changes, and the psychological stresses of new parenthood, but the exact cause is not yet a scientific fact. What is known is how common the blues are, and how upsetting they can be to women who have experienced the crash from elation to unhappiness. Sometimes the crash can come while the woman is still in the hospital. One mother, after the birth of her third child, recalls crying because her husband suggested she eat lunch and she just wasn't hungry. "Minor things would set me off into tears, things that normally wouldn't bother me." Kathryn still remembers vividly being in the hospital with her first child, who was screaming nonstop while she was trying without success to comfort him. She picked him up, patted him on the back, and tried to burp him, but the screaming continued. A friend of hers who is a mother of two then visited her and picked up the baby and soothed him. Finally there was quiet—but that did nothing to soothe Kathryn. When her friend left the room, *she* started crying where her baby had left off. She thought, "Oh my God, she's a good mother and I'm not." She thought of herself as a failure, and she couldn't stop crying.

The blues sometimes hold off until the new family is settled at home. Everything seems to be going fine—and then the tears come. That's what happened to this new mother of a baby girl: "It first happened to me while I was nursing. Just as the baby was about to drift off, my husband put the radio on. I got so angry about it, and felt so oppressed, I screamed at him, 'How can you do that? Turn that thing off!' As I said it I realized how ridiculous it was, and then I cried over my inordinate reaction. Generally I'm not a big crier. This seemed almost like a physiological reaction. I felt vulnerable with fatigue, and out of control. Both my husband and I were taken by surprise by it." Sometimes the husband is the first to notice. His wife just isn't herself, and he can't understand the change in her moods. One new father relates how his wife now cries at the slightest thing. "She's happy and then she's sad. Usually there has to be a death in the family for her to cry. But now she cries a lot, and then gets angry at herself for doing it."

There really is no cause for either self-recrimination or for undue concern. The "blues" are almost an inevitable part of the post-partum period, but not a long-lasting part. They generally go as fast as they come, lasting anywhere from an hour or two to a few days. The best way to deal with them is to simply accept them, to let yourself go through them, to let yourself cry. It's almost as if they balance off the earlier euphoria of the childbirth experience and leave you at a more stable emotional level, ready to cope with your new responsibilities.

But there may be reason for concern if the "blues" don't go away within a few days, or if there's a lot more to them than some crying jags. Women who become suspicious, or confused, or incoherent, or who remain depressed for weeks, should consult with their physicians. They may need counseling or more intensive treatment to deal with their problems. Women who get more than the "blues" after childbirth, who sink into a real depression, often have tendencies toward depression that may have surfaced at other times in their lives. Dr. Barbara Gordon, New York City psychiatrist, traces their problems to their own mothering: "Some people become depressed who have had poor mothers, and then feel ambivalent about their own mothering abilities. Here they are, faced with a child and the constancy of its demands, someone who can only articulate its needs through crying, someone who won't listen when you request them to stop crying, someone you just can't control. There is no end to its needs, and your time is no longer your own. In such a stressful situation, we fall back on our unconscious models, often our role models from childhood, our mothers. But if they were inadequate, or nonresponsive, a woman will often function in the same way with her child. Other women will get depressed because they feel helpless or out of control with so many demands on them, such as I have enumerated."

Dr. Gordon advises depressed women to get help, both for their own good and for their child's. Prolonged depression will interfere with a woman's emotional interaction with her child, and make the child feel rejected and perhaps depressed as well. Psychotherapy can help a woman to undestand the roots of her feelings, to deal with her hostility, sadness and helplessness, and to derive the most emotional satisfaction from the mothering experience. Dr. Gordon also stresses the importance of support groups during this early mothering period, for all women but especially for a woman who tends toward depression. By getting together with other new mothers, she sees that she is not the only woman perplexed by new parenthood and unsure of her mothering abilities, nor is hers the only baby who doesn't sleep, eat, and quiet down on command. She learns, through the ideas and example of these other women, more about what good mothering is about, perhaps more than she learned from her own mother. With those role models to draw from, she can settle more comfortably into her own new motherhood.

In some rare cases, counseling and support groups are not enough to alleviate emotional distress. Some women become so depressed within three months of the delivery that they are considered psychotic, and may be hospitalized and treated with medication and psychotherapy. Fortunately, this is unusual, affecting about 1 in 500 new mothers. As is the case with the much less serious "blues," its cause is not completely understood, but many psychiatrists believe it occurs most commonly in women with a personal or family history of an affective disorder (such as depression or manic-depression). Postpartum depression is a disorder that can be treated successfully, and these women can and very often do go on to become perfectly good mothers. And if they become mothers again, the chances are great—80 to 90%—that they will not suffer a repetition of this early difficult period.

The Early Days

While a small proportion of women do suffer from extreme depression following delivery, for most new mothers it is a time of mixed emotions. It is certainly a time when emotions reign—emotions of elation, of anxiety, of contentment, of confusion. After their short bout with the "blues" many new mothers begin to feel the excitement all over again, the euphoria of creation, the profound joy of ushering a child into the world and announcing to all your world the birth of your baby. You have graduated into parenthood, and you begin to look around at all your fellow graduates. As one new father put it, "I'm now a member of an enormous club of people. Everyone who's ever been a parent is in it. Yet it's also a very exclusive club. I didn't understand the membership qualifications until I was admitted." As a member of this club the rules of your life will be different and the focus of your life will change, at least for a time, to the newest member of your family. You may find that what interested you before seems banal now, that nothing can compete with your latest little love. Danielle, the new mother of twin sons, was astonished at how her babies so completely won her over from her previous passion. "Normally, at this time of the year, I can be found in Saks or in Bloomingdale's or walking down Fifth Avenue buying a lot of stuff I don't need. It's time for sales, and usually I try not to miss any. But this year is different. I haven't seen the inside of a store. That just shows you that my head is not there. My head is here, at home, with my babies."

The joys of this period cannot be matched, the joy of marveling over the miracle of your child, the joys of assuming the mantle of motherhood and knowing that the words "ma-ma" will soon be yours to hear and to savor. You've joined the club, and for now at least you're the star. But along with the benefits of membership there are also some dues to pay—dues that make some new parents wonder just what they got themselves into, and even wish that they hadn't. There's no doubt but that the early weeks of parenthood are difficult and stressful; they've even been described as grueling, and that's hardly an overstatement. While your own body is still in physical flux, you'll be faced with the physical changes your baby is going through in its adjustment from the womb to the world. A newborn baby is biologically disorganized for a time, its bodily systems in transition, its rhythms fluctuating and unpredictable. When it will be sleepy, when it will be hungry, when it will be alert, or irritable, or quietly content, is anybody's guess. What its cries mean and how to stop them seem to be well-kept secrets. The baby's unpredictability can be frustrating, its endless demands exhausting. Even the most patient of parents can begin to feel resentful and to wish, fleetingly, to be free of the burden of this helpless infant. Where are the rewards, you may wonder, as you wait in vain for a smile or for a flicker of recognition from a baby too young to show it.

The frustration can be compounded by physical exhaustion. Sleep deprivation is a reality of the early parenthood period. Newborns don't know night from day, and may not know enough to sleep for more than two hours at a time. No sooner do you set them down than they seem to be up again, crying for food, or attention, or whatever else babies cry for. There may not seem to be much time left over for you to get sleep of your own, or to do much of anything else. June is a mother who was surprised at how little time the baby left her: "I would feed her, put her to sleep, take a shower, and then dry my hair. Halfway through the baby would be up again, so I'd have to go through the day with drippy, droopy hair. When my husband came home at night he would ask, 'What did you do today?' I'd say, 'Oh, at three P.M. I brushed my teeth.' Newcomers wonder just how much time a little baby can take. The answer is it can take *all* your time."

All new babies are demanding, but some are more demanding than others, and their parents assume that they are somehow at fault. Why does their baby cry more than other babies, and sleep less, and seem so inconsolable? Such early differences are a result of a baby's inborn nature, not a reflection on its parents' abilities, but some parents don't see it that way. If only they were better parents their babies would be better babies . . . or so their thinking goes. Feeling inadequate, they may lose their confidence, and actually become less responsive to their baby's needs.

As a mother's life centers on her new baby, she may lose touch with other parts of her life, with the larger world outside her own new world. She may not find the time to read a newspaper or a book, or even feel like doing it if she has the opportunity. The world of work seems worlds away, her old friends to be out of touch with her new reality. So she may feel cut off, isolated, going through an almost universal experience, but going through it alone.

There is no way to eliminate all the stresses of your first weeks with your baby, to feel perfectly calm in your new role, perfectly content with your lot. The very transition into motherhood brings with it stress, as does the sudden and complete responsibility for another human life. But there are ways in which you can minimize the psychic wear and tear, ways we enumerate here, ways that can help get you through the early days without wishing them away.

- *Don't expect miracles*. Taking care of a newborn baby is not all sweetness and light. You'll be tired and frustrated. The baby will be finicky and fretful. Certainly, there will be moments of serenity, when you'll feel at peace with your child, but more often you'll feel in a state of siege. You may have been told that your life will go on as always, that you'll just take your baby along with you wherever you go, that motherhood is no big deal. One pregnant woman, in the beginning stages of decorating her home, expected the infancy period to bring with it no delay in the completion of her new decor. She figured she'd just zip the baby into a baby carrier, flip it on her back, and go right on with her swatch-selecting and color-coordinating. That's the same mother who later found herself going around with wet hair and unbrushed teeth—and a still unfurnished apartment. If you expect the early weeks of motherhood to be easy, you'll be disappointed. If you expect them to be rough, you'll be better prepared for the realities, and grateful for the quiet times that occasionally do punctuate the madness.
- *Don't take it personally*. Your baby isn't crying because you're its mother. Nor is your baby crying to punish you. It is simply in a baby's nature to cry, and in some babies' natures to be colicky, and in some to be poor sleepers, and in some to be poor eaters. It doesn't mean that you're a bad mother. It means that that's the way your baby is. And if you do make a mistake—if you feed the baby too fast and he spits up, if you don't burp her enough and she gets gassy—that doesn't meant you're a bad mother, either. It simply means that you have to learn to be a mother, as we all do. Mothering is not an inherited skill, nor is it a taught skill in this society. It is largely a matter of on-the-job training, and you're going to get plenty of that.
- *Set priorities*. Now is not the time to prepare your home for the white glove test, no matter the visitors who will be trooping through to meet the newest member of the family. Nor is it the time to entertain your guests lavishly, to demonstrate your latest gourmet accomplishment, or even to enhance your reputation as a whiz with spaghetti. As far as the dirt is concerned, it's time for covering up and sweeping under; as far as the food goes, it's time for ordering in.

To be fair to yourself, your baby, and the rest of your family, it's important to conserve your energy for the things that matter most. Your home will still be there, even if it's not as orderly as always. And if your guests, left hungry or unhappy with a pizza dinner, don't come back so soon, that's all the better for you and your need for rest.

You may have heard this advice elsewhere, but it bears repeating: When your baby naps, don't whip out the cooking utensils or cleaning equipment; instead, take a nap if at all possible. Women who have never before been able to sleep during the day discover how easily it comes—and how wonderful it feels—once a new baby is on the scene. You may even find the time to get some of the housework done if you heed this other piece of advice: When your baby is awake, hitch her to you with a baby carrier and go about your household chores. She'll be happy with the closeness and the movement. You'll be happy with the wrinkles you iron out and the clutter you straighten out. And you'll both be happy to be together.

• *Get a babysitter.* Togetherness can be wonderful, but it's got to have its limits. One way is to hire a babysitter an afternoon or two a week while you stay in the house. Getting out is wonderful, too, as we'll discuss soon, but being a free woman in your own home can be an even bigger treat. Someone *else* will change the baby; someone *else* will comfort the baby; you'll be at your leisure to do whatever it is that catches your fancy. It may be doing some part-time work. It may be washing and drying your hair without the fear of interruption. It may just be doing nothing, absolutely nothing. You are not the only one who can care for your baby, but you are the only one who can make sure that your own needs are taken care of.

Hiring a caretaker is particularly important for women who intend to return soon to work outside the home. When the baby is as young as a week or two, the babysitter should start on a schedule of a half a day or a day a week, and then gradually increase it. In that way the baby and the babysitter will get used to each other, and you'll get used to trusting someone else with the baby's care. Many women choose to ease into work as well, starting out part-time, if possible, and gradually extending their hours at the office. Gradual changes are best for you and your baby.

- *Get away.* Getting out of the house is an important diversion for a new mother. Sometimes you'll want to make it a mother-baby trip, whether to sit in the park a spell, visit a museum, perhaps even visit your workplace to show everybody exactly who it is that is keeping you away from the office. But getting out by yourself, or with other adults, is also important in keeping up your spirits. It can remind you that there is a world out there beyond diapers and pacifiers, and that you are more than a mother. But strangely enough, a woman who is eager to get out of the house and away from her child may be just as eager to get back. It's very common for a new mother to miss her baby even during a brief absence. This person who is so new to her life has already won her heart. Parting, even for a short time, can make that very clear to you and will perhaps make some of the more demanding aspects of your baby's care easier for you to take.

- *Join a group.* As you enter new motherhood, you may find that some of your points of common interest with your old friends are gone. You may begin to feel alienated from your old support systems, particularly ones at work. You may not even have realized how much support your professional colleagues and the structure of your work provided you. But now that it's gone, if only temporarily, you may keenly feel its lack. Who's going to give you the praise and respect now that was an integral part of your working life? Who's going to comment on your competency in mothering? Certainly not the person being mothered. The baby is too busy being a baby to take note of how good a mother you're becoming. This lack of acknowledgment, especially to a woman used to receiving daily acknowledgment for her professional accomplishments, can produce feelings of isolation and inadequacy. The way to combat those feelings is to join a new support group, a group of new mothers who are going through the same experiences you are, a group that can support both your feelings and your actions.

A support group, vital to women who tend toward depression, also serves important functions for the average, harried mother of a newborn. It provides reinforcement for your mothering techniques, as well as ideas for improving them, or at least for doing them faster. It provides the reassurance that other women are experiencing the same range of emotions you are, including the sometimes uncomfortable one of resenting the baby, even of momentarily regretting its birth. For you to hear other women admitting it is to know that you're normal, and not evil, for your feeling. Discussing such negative emotions also provides a good safety valve, a way to keep them from being acted out. On its most basic level, a group of new mothers provides the company that many women in this position crave. It helps them to stave off the loneliness that can pervade this child-focused period, the isolation that is the lot of many new mothers. Some women have a built-in support system in their friends who have had babies at about the same time they did. Others have to work a little bit harder at it, ideally beginning before the baby is born. Perhaps you can connect up to women in your childbirth preparation course, and plan to meet on an ongoing basis both before and after the babies are on the scene. Or you may spot other equally pregnant women around the neighborhood, and use your common state to strike up a conversation, and perhaps later even a friendship. Early motherhood is a busy time, but it's not too busy to gather together a group of women so you can acknowledge your mutual strengths, and even have some laughs while you're doing it.

- *This too shall pass.* The early period of motherhood is so consuming that it may seem as if it will never end. But it will, before you even know it. The baby who awakened every two hours will start sleeping for three-hour stretches, and then four. One morning you'll wake up and be surprised that the morning has come. What happened to the 2:00 A.M. feeding? Is the baby all right? The baby is perfectly fine, just a little more mature and a little less disorganized. With every passing week, life with baby will become less hectic, less exhausting, and less consuming. Parents who can understand that ahead of time will find the hardest of times not quite so trying. One new mother was helped a lot by the comment of a more experienced mother. "She said to me, 'If only I had known how quickly the beginning, unsettled period goes, I would have been more patient.' I kept that in mind. She was right. My baby is twelve weeks old now, and the months really flew by."

The time does fly by, and one day you may look back and think it all went too fast. The mother of an older baby, seven-month-old Jason, was caught by surprise at how far along he'd come. "One day he just took off. He pulled himself up, he started to crawl, he began to climb up the stairs. It all happened at once, and I wasn't really ready for it. I started getting misty thinking, 'My baby's infancy is over.' I really felt badly about it ending."

No, the early days of motherhood aren't easy, but they are an important part of your baby's development and of your growing relationship with him, a part that your baby may finally put behind him more readily than you do.

The Father's Role

You may have noted, so far in this chapter, a puzzling omission in the cast of characters. While much has been said about the baby's behavior, and the mother's responses, the father's input into the new family's dynamics has drawn a blank. Unfortunately, that is a reflection of the way things are in many newly formed families: The mother and the child form a tight bond, while the father remains a shadowy, elusive figure, unable or unwilling to forge his own meaningful bond with his new child. While things are beginning to change for the better, as more and more fathers become involved in new parenthood, there are still forces that work to keep the father on the edge of the new family unit. One is a problem of our society, a society that rarely relaxes its work rules to allow full paternal participation in child-rearing, even in the early, formative months. It's rare for a man to be allowed more than a few weeks' leave after the birth of his child, or for him to be allowed a flexible work schedule so that he can combine his professional life with a meaningful role in his child's life.

The other blocks are also societal ones, but ones that have been internalized by both father and mother. Most of today's adult males have been brought up to believe that child-rearing is women's

work; their own fathers didn't do it, and they don't know how.
"The woman is seen as the primary caretaker," emphasize Doctors
Handler and Kestenbaum, New York psychotherapists. "The baby
emerges from her. Her breasts fill up with milk to feed it. And
the child begins to gravitate toward her. The father often feels
disconnected to the child because the child doesn't come to him
in the same kind of way. But this is partly a function of his own
passivity. Many men are reluctant to take a more active stand and
to inject themselves into their child's life in a meaningful way.
They often relate to the child through the mother, not through
their own active efforts to engage the child in a relationship of
their own."

The mother can contribute to the father's "outsider" status by
treating the baby as her own personal property, as belonging to
her and to her alone. Although she may give lip service to encouraging her husband's involvement, she may really undermine
his every effort, criticizing the way he holds the bottle and holds
the baby, whisking the infant away at the earliest opportunity. One
man said he learned to stay away because his wife expressed guilt
every time he tended the baby. But this kind of attitude cheats
not only the father and the child, it cheats the mother as well. Her
possessiveness may spark jealousy in her husband—a jealousy that
will backfire on the marital relationship. He'll be jealous of the
special bond that his wife and baby share, and angry at his wife
for being more available to the baby than to him.

In some families, the scenario is a little different; it is the wife
who is jealous of her husband's involvement with the baby, fearful
that the baby will favor him over her. She is the one who feels
excluded. Wherever there is this kind of rivalry for the baby and
for each other, instead of a shared commitment to the family as
a loving, growing unit, there is likely to be marital dissension. This
tension may be compounded by other realities of the newborn
period: the exhaustion engendered by sleep deprivation; the in-
securities of being new parents; the stress created by a new way
of life; the prohibition of sex for a time, and then the awkwardness
or the pain upon first resuming it again. And then there is the
question of just how to parent this new person in your lives: Should
the baby be left to "cry it out," or picked up and comforted to
quiet it down? Should it be fed by breast or by bottle, by demand
or by schedule? The questions can seem infinite in number, and

infinitely difficult for parents to agree upon. And you may begin
to ask yourself the question: Can this marriage be saved?

The answer is that it can not only be saved, but enhanced, if
the groundwork is laid before the baby's birth. Some couples say
that new parenthood brings them closer together than ever. Says
one father of a newborn, "My relationship with my wife has less
of a negative side now. We have occasional arguments, but we
fight less than we usually do. There is more caring on both our
parts." To achieve such harmony, questions of child-care philosophy should be discussed during the pregnancy, and differences
ironed out. Mates who have become practiced at the art of compromise will find that it stands them in good stead when it comes
to child-rearing issues. One decision some women make ahead of
time, with their husbands and marriages in mind, is not to breast-
feed their babies. They fear that their husbands will feel left out
and uninvolved, and will choose to stay that way. But research has
proven that fear unfounded. According to a recent study of new
parents, the husbands of breast-feeding women enjoyed their newborn infants even more than did the husbands of bottle-feeders,
and they engaged the babies in more activity. If a husband does
feel "left out" on that score, he can be given the job of providing
the baby with a nightly relief bottle. More likely he'll be satisfied
with all the *other* things he can do for the baby—the bathing, the
dressing, the cuddling—and will be happy to leave the feeding to
you.

Some couples divide the baby care chores—with the mother
responsible for feeding, for example, and father in charge of bathing—while others divvy up the day or the evening into time slots,
such as alternating responsibility every two hours. By explicitly
delegating responsibility, they find that they avoid constant arguing
about who should be doing what, when. Other couples find that
a less structured division of labor works better. Reports the father
of a four-month-old son, "My wife and I have a give-and-take
relationship. Certain things she does, certain things I do. Certain
things neither of us likes to do, but somehow they get done. We
have no laundry list. It's not 'This is your job, this is mine.' It's
catch as catch can. For us, it works out very well."

Once your baby is born, your challenge will be to allow your
husband more of a role with your child so that they can develop
a comfortable relationship. If you show him that you welcome his

help, if you share the new experience with him rather than shelter him from it, your baby is more likely to have an active, participating father. Not only will they be happier with each other, you'll be happier and more confident when you want to get out of the house and leave your husband in charge. It's never too soon to give your husband a chance at primary caretaking, but if you wait a number of months, it can seem as if it's too late. That's what happened to Caroline, a 40-year-old psychotherapist who waited almost two months before going out one evening to the office and leaving her husband and baby alone. "I was so happy to get out and back to work. Little did I know what was happening in my absence. My husband was so scared, and the baby wouldn't take the relief bottle he offered her. It was a horrible first experience for them both. When I walked back into the house the baby was screaming. The first thing my husband said was 'Thank God you're here,' and then he started ranting and raving that I should have hired a babysitter, that he's too tired at night to take care of her. I was furious. 'My God,' I thought, 'he's the child's father. If he can't cope and soothe her, how can hired help do it?' I was momentarily frightened that I would never be able to leave again, that this was the end of my separate professional life. But then we talked a lot about it. We discussed the problems and our feelings, and we even talked it over with the pediatrician. As one solution, we decided that my husband should take on more of the parenting chores, even when I'm home. The second time I left him and the baby together they were fine. It probably was because he wasn't as anxious. He was calmer and more able to soothe the baby. When I walked in everything was quiet and peaceful. He had gotten in touch with himself as a father."

Caroline and her husband did exactly the right thing when they decided to talk, not fight. During this period, there'll be a lot to talk about, as emotional issues come up for both parents. It's not just the mother who is prone to stress and depression. Research has shown that fathers are also vulnerable to depression after the birth of a baby. As you recall, they may have gotten through the pregnancy quite calmly, but the postpartum days are likely to be a different story. *This* is when the reality hits them. *This* is when they are first faced with having a baby, and being a father. As Doctors Handler and Kestenbaum point out, "The storm is greater for the father after the baby is born. This is when he is more conscious of rumblings within himself, and more willing to explore. It is also a good time for his wife to give some mothering to him, and to make room for him to explore his own motherliness. Together, they form a partnership, each giving when the other most needs it."

The giving can be done in different ways. It can be done by spending time alone with your husband, even when there doesn't seem to be enough time in the day. Hiring a babysitter and going out as a couple will help you to keep your relationship fresh and growing, and your baby will survive your absence. The giving can be done by giving together to the baby, by sometimes bathing her together, playing with her together, enjoying together the life you created in unison. It can be done by making an effort to do it, although sometimes it can seem like too much of an effort to bother. Ellen is a woman who has done it three times now, and found that it's paid off: "After each of the three children were born, I've been very, very tired. Jeff has wanted to stay up at night and do things. I've just wanted to crash. But I knew I just couldn't die on him night after night. I knew you have to try to be your charming, romantic, scintillating self at least some of the time. It's worked for us. We're still married, and we're happy together." That doesn't mean jumping into your husband's arms when you're aching with exhaustion, or serving a candlelit dinner as you hear your baby crying for food or for attention. It does mean that your husband needs attention, too, and that while you are certainly busy being a new mother, it's no time to stop being a mate.

Although the suggestions given in this past section apply to everyone, it seems that many "older" parents have been doing quite well on their own. A study recently conducted by two California psychiatrists found that older fathers were more involved in the parenting role than were younger ones. Interviewed after the birth of the first child, they generally expressed enjoyment in parenting, spent considerable time with their children, and were better able to integrate work and family responsibilities. According to a 34-year-old new father, who is married to an "older" woman of 38, "It's so exciting dealing with a child at this stage. It's fascinating to watch him go through fundamental changes and growth and development. Some fathers underplay it. They say they're proud they never changed a diaper or gave the baby a bath. But men my age have a different sense of maturity. They have less fear in dealing with the baby. They don't want to miss out."

The same study also made some positive findings about so-called "late" mothers (who averaged 36 in age). Among the advantages it found were greater maturity, an enhanced sense of competence, and an emphasis on the creative and pleasurable aspects of parenthood. Even in a comparison between older working mothers and younger ones, the older mothers excelled. They "seemed to divide their time more comfortably between their children and their social and professional lives and to be less resentful of their children's demands," reported Doctors Steven Frankel and Myra Wise in the journal *Psychiatry*. "In short, they were more likely to be satisfied with their situation, in spite of the stresses involved, and to meet the criteria set forth in the literature for succeeding as a parent while working outside the home." To older parents, working or not, "a baby may be seen as a commitment to the future and a meaningful opportunity to recreate the family."

When you're awakened from your slumber by the cry of your hungry baby, when you spend your nights rocking her to try to get her to sleep, you may question those results. You may wonder whether you've waited too long, whether your best years are behind you, whether you're simply too old for this baby business. But as the days and weeks go by, as your baby smiles at you and reaches out for your love, you'll realize that you've waited just long enough. This is the baby you've been waiting for, and for your whole new family, the best is yet to come.

Index

About the Authors

Dr. Kathryn Schrotenboer has a full-time obstetrics and gynecology practice in Manhattan, where many of her patients are over 35. She is an attending physician at the New York Hospital/Cornell Medical Center. She has a regular column in *Family Circle* magazine. Dr. Schrotenboer lives with her son and twin daughters in New York.

Joan Solomon Weiss has written for *Ms.*, *The Washington Post*, *Vogue*, and *Science Digest*. She is the winner of the prestigious Howard W. Blakeslee Award, sponsored by the American Heart Association. The author of *Your Second Child* (Summit Books), she lives with her husband and two small children in New York.